Current Topics in Microbiology and Immunology

Volume 401

More information about this series at http://www.springer.com/series/82

Kazuichi Okazaki
Editor

IgG4-Related Disease

Responsible Series Editor: Tasuku Honjo

Springer

Editor
Kazuichi Okazaki
Department of Gastroenterology and
Hepatology
Kansai Medical University
Osaka
Japan

ISSN 0070-217X ISSN 2196-9965 (electronic)
Current Topics in Microbiology and Immunology
ISBN 978-3-319-52541-9 ISBN 978-3-319-52542-6 (eBook)
DOI 10.1007/978-3-319-52542-6

Library of Congress Control Number: 2017934518

Printed on acid-free paper

This Springer imprint is published by Springer Nature
The registered company is Springer International Publishing AG
The registered company address is: Gewerbestrasse 11, 6330 Cham, Switzerland

Preface

IgG4-related disease (IgG4-RD) is a novel clinical entity, originally proposed from Japan and has been worldwide accepted. According to recognizing the disease concept, novel nomenclatures for IgG4-related conditions in individual organs have been proposed. Although the pathogenesis and pathophysiology of IgG4-RD still remain unclear, recent studies have suggested abnormal innate/acquired immunity based on immunogenic backgrounds. This volume consists of nine chapters focusing on recent progress in the pathogenesis and pathophysiology of IgG4-RD in addition to the disease concept, diagnosis and treatment. Readers can understand this novel clinical entity well, and recent progress in the pathogenesis and pathophysiology of IgG4-RD.

Osaka, Japan Kazuichi Okazaki

Contents

Current Concept of IgG4-Related Disease

Kazuichi Okazaki and Hisanori Umehara

Abstract IgG4-related disease (IgG4-RD) is a fibroinflammatory disease of unknown etiology, which is characterized by a tendency to form tumefactive lesions, increased serum levels of IgG4, and massive infiltration of IgG4-positive plasma cells with storiform fibrosis and/or obliterative phlebitis. Patients with IgG4-RD have frequently multiorgan involvements such as the pancreas, biliary tree, salivary glands, periorbital tissues, kidneys, lungs, lymph nodes, and retroperitoneum. IgG4-RD mainly affects middle-aged to elderly men except for involvement in lachrymal and salivary glands, so-called Mikulicz's disease. The clinical manifestations of IgG4-RD depend on individually involved organs and respond well to steroid, but the prognosis still remains unclear. Some patients develop serious complications such as obstructive jaundice due to hepatic, gall-bladder, or pancreatic lesions; hydronephrosis due to retroperitoneal fibrosis; or respiratory symptoms due to pulmonary lesions. Nomenclatures of individual organ manifestation of IgG4-RD have been internationally consented.

Abbreviations

AIP	Autoimmune pancreatitis
CDC	Comprehensive diagnostic criteria
GEL	Granulocytic epithelial lesion
ICDC	International consensus diagnostic criteria
IDCP	Idiopathic duct-centric pancreatitis
IgG4-RD	IgG4-related disease
IgG4-SC	IgG4-related sclerosing cholangitis

K. Okazaki
Department of Gastroenterology and Hepatology, Kansai Medical University, Osaka, Japan

K. Okazaki (✉)
The Third Department of Internal Medicine, Division of Gastroenterology and Hepatology, Kansai Medical University, Shinmachi, Hirakata, Osaka 573-1197, Japan
e-mail: okazaki@hirakata.kmu.ac.jp

H. Umehara
Northern County Center for RA and Autoimmune Disease, Hayashi Hospital, Fukui, Japan

Current Topics in Microbiology and Immunology (2017) 401: 1–18
DOI 10.1007/82_2016_47

Published Online: 26 December 2016

IPC	The international pathologic consensus criteria
JPS	Japan Pancreas Society
LPSP	Lymphoplasmacytic sclerosing pancreatitis
MD	Mikulicz's disease
MOLPS	Multiorgan lymphoproliferative disease
OOI	Other organ involvement
SjS	SJÖGREN'S syndrome
PSC	Primary sclerosing cholangitis
RF	Rheumatoid factor
SIPS	Systemic IgG4-related plasmacytic syndrome

Contents

1 The History of IgG4-Related Disease: Before and After Discovery of IgG4 (Table 1)

IgG4-related disease (IgG4-RD) is a fibroinflammatory disease recognized as a novel clinical entity with multiorgan involvement and unknown origin, associated with abundant infiltration of IgG4-positive cells (Kamisawa and Okamoto 2006; Yamamoto et al. 2006; Masaki et al. 2009; Umehara et al. 2012a, b; Deshpande et al. 2012; Stone et al. 2012; Okazaki et al. 2011). IgG4-RD has been found to affect the pancreas (Hamano et al. 2001; Okazaki et al. 2009), bile duct (Okazaki et al. 2009; Nakazawa et al. 2001), lachrymal glands (Okazaki et al. 2009; Kamisawa et al. 2003), salivary glands (Okazaki et al. 2009; Kamisawa et al. 2003), central nervous system (Okazaki et al. 2009; Kishimoto et al. 2000; Shimatsu et al. 2009), thyroid (Okazaki et al. 2009; Komatsu et al. 2005; Li et al. 2010), lung

Table 1 History of IgG4-related disease

Authors (year)	Evidences/Contents
Mikulicz et al. (1892)	Mikulicz's disease (*Z. Chir. Fesrschr*)
Sarles et al. (1961)	Hypergammaglobulinemia in CP (*Am J Dig Di*)
Comings et al. (1967)	Familial multifocal fibrosclerosis (*Ann Intern Med*)
Küttner (1972)	Küttner tumor (*Acta Otolaryngol*)
Kawaguchi et al. (1991)	Lymphoplasmacytic sclerosing pancreatitis (*Human Pathol*)
Yoshida et al. (1995)	Autoimmune pancreatitis (*Dig Dis Sci*)
Hamano et al. (2001)	High IgG4 levels in sclerosing pancretitis (*N Eng J Med*)
Japan Pancreas Society (2002)	Clinical diagnostic criteria for AIP 200 (*Suizo*)
Okazaki et al. (2006)	Clinical diagnostic criteria for AIP 2006 (*J Gastroenterol*)
Chari et al. (2006)	Mayo criteria (*Clin Gastroenterol Hepatol*)
Kamisawa et al. (2006)	IgG4-related sclerosing disease (*J Gastroenterol*)
Yamamoto et al. (2006)	IgG4-related plasmacytic disease (*Mod Rheumatol*)
Masaki et al. (2009)	IgG4-multiorgan lymphoproliferative syndrome (MOLPS) (*Ann Rheum Dis*)
Shimosegawa et al. (2011)	International Consensus Diagnostic Criteria (ICDC) for AIP (*Pancreas*)
Umehara et al. (2012)	Concept and comprehensive diagnostic criteria for IgG4-related disease (*Mod Rheumatol*)
Deshpande et al. (2012)	International Pathological Consensus for IgG4-RD (*Mod Pathol*)
Stone et al. (2012)	Nomenclatures of individual organ manifestation of IgG4-RD (*Arthritis Rheum*)

(Okazaki et al. 2009; Zen et al. 2009; Matsui et al. 2012), liver (Okazaki et al. 2009; Umemura et al. 2007; Umemura et al. 2011), gastrointestinal tract (Okazaki et al. 2009; Lopes et al. 2010; Uehara et al. 2010; Ravi et al. 2009; Ueno et al. 2008), kidney (Okazaki et al. 2009; Uchiyama-Tanaka et al. 2004; Takeda et al. 2004), prostate (Okazaki et al. 2009; Yoshimura et al. 2006; Nishimori et al. 2007), retroperitoneum (Okazaki et al. 2009; Hamano et al. 2002), arteries (Okazaki et al. 2009; Stone et al. 2009), lymph nodes (Okazaki et al. 2009; Saegusa et al. 2003), skin (Okazaki et al. 2009; Sato et al. 2012), and breast (Okazaki et al. 2009; Cheuk et al. 2009). However, before the disease was identified, each organ lesion was described independently.

In 1892, Mikulicz (1892) first observed a patient with symmetrical swelling of the lachrymal, parotid, and submandibular glands, with massive infiltration of mononuclear cells. The condition was called Mikulicz's disease (MD); however, it has since been classified as an atypical type of Sjögren's syndrome, which also presents with bilateral, painless, and symmetrical swelling of the lachrymal, parotid, and submandibular glands. Küttner reported a tumor-like enlargement of the submandibular gland that was sometimes a result of stones in the Wharton duct (Küttner 1896), which indicated that the underlying cause had not been identified. In 1961, Sarles et al. (1961) first observed a case of particular pancreatitis with hypergammaglobulinemia, a prototype of autoimmune pancreatitis (AIP). The concept of AIP was first proposed by Yoshida et al. (1995). Following the histopathological description of lymphoplasmacytic sclerosing pancreatitis (LPSP) in 1991, from the resected pancreas of tumor-forming pancreatitis, which are clinically difficult to distinguish from pancreatic cancer, has been regarded as a characteristic histopathological finding of IgG4-related AIP (type 1 AIP) (Kawaguchi et al. 1991). In 1967, Comings et al. (1967) reported the first familiar case of multifocal fibrosclerosis with retroperitoneal fibrosis, mediastinal fibrosis, sclerosing cholangitis, Riedel's thyroiditis, and pseudotumor of the orbit, which is now regarded as the synonym of IgG4-RD.

Hamano et al. (2001) reported increased serum levels of IgG4 in Japanese patients with AIP, an epoch-making discovery in the history of IgG4-RD. Thereafter, many studies of AIP have been reported, mainly by Japanese investigators. The histopathological findings of LPSP are characterized by the periductal localization of predominantly CD4-positive T cells, IgG4-positive plasma cells, storiform fibrosis with acinar cell atrophy frequently resulting in stenosis of the main pancreatic duct, and obliterative fibrosis (Okazaki et al. 2009). About 60–80 % of patients with AIP show obstructive jaundice with sclerosing cholangitis (IgG4-related sclerosing cholangitis; IgG4-SC) and other organ involvement (OOI), in which cholangiographic features are similar to those of primary sclerosing cholangitis (PSC), pancreatic cancer, and cholangiocarcinoma. The steroid responses and the prognoses of sclerosing cholangitis associated with AIP differ from patients with PSC, which suggests different pathological conditions. In 2003, Kamisawa et al. (2003) suggested that AIP is a systemic sclerosing disease. This was based on the findings that the pancreas and other involved organs have fibrosis with abundant infiltration of IgG4-positive plasma cells. This is similar to the concept of multifocal fibrosclerosis proposed by Comings et al. (1967). Further histological and clinical profiling of patients with "AIP" reveals two distinct subtypes, type 1 and type 2 (Chari et al. 2010; Shimosegawa et al. 2011). Type 1 AIP is classified as a pancreatic manifestation of IgG4-RD and is probably a systemic disease with an abnormal immunological process. Type 2 AIP is thought to be a specific pancreatic disease with granulocytic epithelial lesion (GEL) (Notohara et al. 2003; Zamboni et al. 2004) and occasional coexistence with ulcerative colitis (Shimosegawa et al. 2011; Klöppel et al. 2010).

Conversely, most patients with MD show elevated serum levels of IgG4, negative anti-SS-A/Ro or anti-SS-B/La antibodies, infiltration of IgG4-positive plasma cells into the glands, and recovery of secretion with steroid treatment. The patients with MD often show steroid-responsive OOIs such as AIP, sclerosing cholangitis, retroperitoneal fibrosis, enlarged celiac and hilar lymph nodes, chronic thyroiditis, or interstitial nephritis (Kamisawa and Okamoto 2006; Yamamoto et al. 2006; Masaki et al. 2009; Umehara et al. 2012a, b; Okazaki et al. 2009). MD has been considered to be completely different from Sjögren's syndrome because of its responsiveness to steroid treatment (Kamisawa and Okamoto 2006; Yamamoto et al. 2006; Masaki et al. 2009; Umehara et al. 2012a, b; Okazaki et al. 2009).

In addition to the original concept of multifocal idiopathic fibrosclerosis, recent studies led us to develop a novel concept of a systemic disease such as IgG4-related systemic sclerosing disease (Kamisawa and Okamoto 2006), systemic IgG4-related plasmacytic syndrome (SIPS) (Yamamoto et al. 2006), or IgG4-positive multiorgan lymphoproliferative syndrome (IgG4-MOLPS) (Masaki et al. 2009), all of which may refer to the same conditions. Based on these findings, the members of the Japanese Research Committees for "Systemic IgG4-related Sclerosing Disease" (chaired by Professor Okazaki) and "IgG4-MOLPS" (chaired by Professor Umehara), both of which were supported by the Research for Intractable Disease Program from the Ministry of Health, Labor and Welfare of Japan, have agreed that the comprehensive term "IgG4-related disease (IgG4-RD)" includes these conditions at a minimum, although pathogenesis and pathophysiology remain unclear (Umehara et al. 2012a, b). The first International Symposium on IgG4-RD held in Boston (chaired by Professor Stone of Massachusetts General Hospital) endorsed the Japanese concept and proposed nomenclatures and pathological criteria for individual organ lesions (Deshpande et al. 2012; Stone et al. 2012).

2 Current Concepts of IgG4-RD

Patients with IgG4-RD show diffuse or focal organ enlargement and mass-forming or nodular/thickened lesions in various organs, either synchronously or metachronously (Figs. 1 and 2). This is due to the prominent infiltration of lymphocytes and plasmacytes with fibrosis (Umehara et al. 2012a). The causes of the disease are still not clear; however, some abnormal immunological mechanisms are involved based on the immunogenic backgrounds. The organs known to be affected include the pancreas, biliary duct, lacrimal/salivary glands, retroperitoneum, central nervous system, thyroid gland, lungs, liver, gastrointestinal tracts, kidneys, prostate, mesenterium, and lymph nodes (Lopes et al. 2010; Uehara et al. 2010; Ravi et al. 2009; Ueno et al. 2008; Uchiyama-Tanaka et al. 2004; Takeda et al. 2004; Yoshimura et al. 2006; Nishimori et al. 2007; Hamano et al. 2002; Stone et al. 2009; Saegusa et al. 2003; Sato et al. 2012; Cheuk et al. 2009; Mikulicz 1892; Küttner 1896; Sarles et al. 1961; Yoshida et al. 1995; Kawaguchi et al. 1991; Comings et al. 1967; Chari et al. 2010; Shimosegawa et al. 2011). IgG4-RD mainly affects middle-aged to elderly men except for the involvement in lachrymal and salivary glands, so-called Mikulicz's disease, in which the previous epidemiological studies did not show gender difference (Yamamoto et al. 2015). Clinical symptoms vary depending on the organ in which the lesions are located and dramatically relieved by steroid therapy in many cases (Kamisawa and Okamoto 2006; Yamamoto et al. 2006; Masaki et al. 2009; Umehara et al. 2012a, b; Deshpande et al. 2012; Stone et al. 2012; Okazaki et al. 2011; Hamano et al. 2001); however,

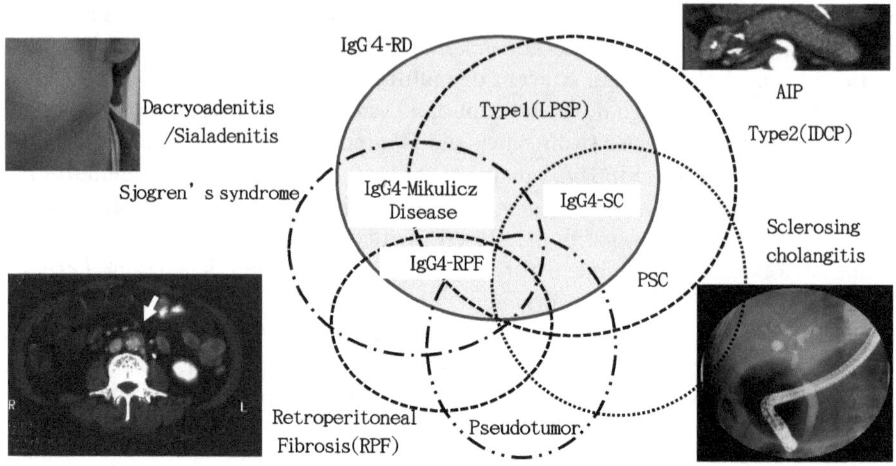

Fig. 1 Current concept of IgG4-related disease (Kamisawa et al. J Gastroenterol 2003; Umehara et al. Mod Rheumatol 2010)

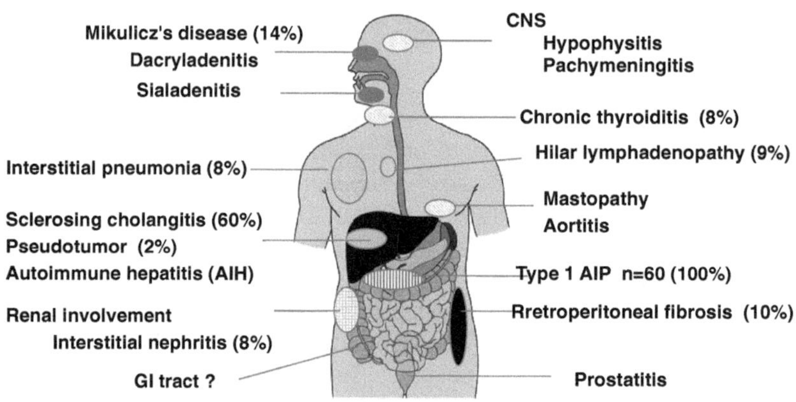

Fig. 2 Other organ involvement (OOIs) in type 1 AIP (Okazaki et al. J Gastroenterol 2008)

the prognosis is not clear. Some patients develop serious complications such as obstructive jaundice due to hepatic, gallbladder, or pancreatic lesions; hydronephrosis due to retroperitoneal fibrosis; or respiratory symptoms due to pulmonary lesions (Kamisawa and Okamoto 2006; Yamamoto et al. 2006; Masaki et al. 2009; Umehara et al. 2012a, b; Deshpande et al. 2012; Stone et al. 2012; Okazaki et al. 2011; Hamano et al. 2001; Okazaki et al. 2009; Uchiyama-Tanaka et al. 2004; Takeda et al. 2004; Hamano et al. 2002). Although the infiltration of IgG4-positive cells and increased serum levels of IgG4 are characteristics in

IgG4-RD, the severity of fibrosis seems to be different among the individual organs involved. These conditions are quite similar to multifocal idiopathic fibrosclerosis (Comings et al. 1967). Storiform fibrosis and obliterative phlebitis are characteristic in most organ involvements including pancreatic, biliary tract, retroperitoneal, and renal lesions, but the degree varies depending on the individual organs. For example, very seldom do lesions appear in the lachrymal/salivary gland or lymph node. The previous nomenclature of "IgG4-related sclerosing disease" (Kamisawa and Okamoto 2006) is mainly based on the fibrous swollen organs, whereas those of "IgG4-SIPS" (Yamamoto et al. 2006) and "IgG4 + MOLPS" (Masaki et al. 2009) have been based on lymphoplasmacytic proliferation and swollen lymph nodes without fibrosis.

Although most patients have multiorgan lesions synchronously or metachronously, about 10–20 % of the patients do not have confirmed other organ involvements (Okazaki et al. 2011). Therefore, it is unclear whether the pathogenic mechanism is same among individual organs or not.

3 Nomenclatures and Individual Organ Manifestation of IgG4-RD

Because multiorgan involvements may occur in IgG4-RD as described above, IgG4-RD includes a wide variety of diseases, including MD, AIP, hypophysitis, Riedel thyroiditis, interstitial pneumonitis, interstitial nephritis, prostatitis, lymphadenopathy, retroperitoneal fibrosis, inflammatory aortic aneurysm, and inflammatory pseudotumor (Kamisawa and Okamoto 2006; Yamamoto et al. 2006; Masaki et al. 2009; Umehara et al. 2012a, b; Deshpande et al. 2012; Stone et al. 2012; Okazaki et al. 2009, 2011; Hamano et al. 2001). In the International Symposium on IgG4-RD, the nomenclature of individual organ manifestations of IgG4-RD were proposed (Table 2) using "IgG4-related" as a modifier, except for the pancreatic manifestation (Stone et al. 2012). The pancreatic manifestation of IgG4-RD was termed "type 1 autoimmune pancreatitis (IgG4-related pancreatitis)." The term "type 1 AIP" is now widely accepted among gastroenterologists and pancreatic surgeons. It also serves to discriminate between type 1 and type 2 AIP, which is not a part of the IgG4-RD spectrum. When the pathogenesis of type 2 AIP is clarified, the term "type 1 AIP" might be replaced by "IgG4-related pancreatitis." In the biliary manifestation, the nomenclature for IgG4-related biliary tract (but not gall bladder) disease includes "sclerosing" to distinguish between the primary and IgG4-related forms of sclerosing cholangitis.

Table 2 Preferred nomenclature for individual organ manifestations of IgG4-related disease (Stone et al. 2012)

Organ system/tissue	Preferred name
Pancreas	Type 1 autoimmune pancreatitis (IgG4-related pancreatitis)
Eye	IgG4-related ophthalmic disease is the general term for the peri-ocular manifestations of this disease. There are several subsets, outlined below
Lacrimal glands	IgG4-related dacryoadenitis
Orbital soft tissue (orbital inflammatory pseudotumor)	IgG4-related orbital inflammation
Extra-ocular muscle disease	IgG4-related orbital myositis
Orbit with involvement of multiple anatomic structures	IgG4-related pan-orbital inflammation (includes lacrimal gland disease, extra-ocular muscle involvement, and other potential intra-orbital complications)
Salivary glands (parotid and submandibular glands)	IgG4-related sialadenitis or, more specifically, IgG4-related parotitis or IgG4-related submandibular gland disease
Pachymeninges	IgG4-related pachymeningitis
Hypophysis	IgG4-related hypophysitis
Thyroid (Riedel's thyroiditis)	IgG4-related thyroid disease
Aorta	IgG4-related aortitis/peri-aortitis
Arteries	IgG4-related periarteritis
Mediastinum	IgG4-related mediastinitis
Retroperitoneum	IgG4-related retroperitoneal fibrosis
Mesentery	IgG4-related mesenteritis
Skin	IgG4-related skin disease
Lymph node	IgG4-related lymphadenopathy
Bile ducts	IgG4-related sclerosing cholangitis
Gallbladder	IgG4-related cholecystitis
Liver	IgG4-related hepatopathy (refers to liver involvement that is distinct from biliary tract involvement)
Lung	IgG4-related lung disease
Pleura	IgG4-related pleuritis
Pericardium	IgG4-related pericarditis
Kidney	IgG4-related kidney disease. The specific renal pattern should be termed IgG4-related tubulointerstitial nephritis and membranous glomerulonephritis secondary to IgG4-RD. Involvement of the renal pelvis should be termed IgG4-related renal pyelitis
Breast	IgG4-related mastitis
Prostate	IgG4-related prostatitis

3.1 *Type 1 Autoimmune Pancreatitis (IgG4-Related Pancreatitis)*

Recent studies have suggested that AIP is classified as two distinct subtypes, types 1 and 2 (Shimosegawa et al. 2011). Clinically, type 1 AIP seems to be the pancreatic manifestation of IgG4RD, which is characterized by the following: (1) mild abdominal symptoms, usually without acute attacks of pancreatitis; (2) occasional occurrence of obstructive jaundice; (3) increased serum gammaglobulin, IgG, and/or IgG4 concentrations; (4) the presence of autoantibodies; (5) diffuse, segmental or focal enlargement of the pancreas with a capsule-like low-density rim on dynamic CT/MRI images; (6) irregular narrowing of the main pancreatic duct on endoscopic retrograde cholangiopancreatography (ERCP) images; (7) histopathologically, lymphoplasmacytic sclerosing pancreatitis (LPSP): abundant infiltration of lymphocytes and IgG4-positive plasmacytes and fibrosis, and obliterative phlebitis; (8) occasional association with extrapancreatic lesions such as sclerosing cholangitis similar to primary sclerosing cholangitis (PSC), cholecystitis, sclerosing sialoadenitis, retroperitoneal fibrosis, interstitial renal tubular disorders, enlarged abdominal and mediastinal lymph nodes, chronic thyroiditis, and pseudotumor of the pancreas, liver, or lung; and (9) responsiveness to steroid therapy. Patients with type 1 AIP often have obstructive jaundice, with both pancreatic and extrapancreatic manifestations responding to steroid therapy (Okazaki et al. 2011; Shimosegawa et al. 2011).

Histological examination by American and European pathologists of the resected pancreases of patients with chronic non-alcoholic pancreatitis revealed another histopathological pattern, called idiopathic duct-centric pancreatitis (IDCP) or AIP with granulocytic epithelial lesions (GELs), later named as type 2 AIP (Notohara et al. 2003; Zamboni et al. 2004). Although patients with type 2 AIP show similar pancreas images to type 1 AIP, they show different clinicopathological features from type 1 AIP such as no elevation of serum IgG4, seldom infiltration of IgG4-positive plasma cells, no autoantibodies, or no involvement of other organs, except for inflammatory bowel disease. The most characteristic feature of type 2 AIP is GEL, commonly accompanied by the destruction and obliteration of the pancreatic duct (Shimosegawa et al. 2011). Although type 1 AIP (LPSP type) often occurs in older men and is accompanied by a variety of extrapancreatic lesions, type 2 AIP (IDCP/GEL type) has no gender difference, younger age at onset (often <40 years), and is frequently associated with inflammatory bowel disease (about 30 %). Thus, after a worldwide debate over the diagnostic criteria for AIP, LPSP has been defined as type 1 (IgG4-related pancreatitis) and IDCP/AIP with GEL has been defined as type 2 (Shimosegawa et al. 2011).

3.2 *IgG4-Related Sclerosing Cholangitis (IgG4-SC)*

Bile duct lesions are frequently associated with AIP. For example, 73 % of patients with AIP have shown wall thickening or sclerosing changes in extrapancreatic bile ducts on endoscopic ultrasonography (EUS) and intraductal ultrasonography (IDUS), though only 26 % of patients with AIP demonstrated sclerosing changes by ERCP (Hamano et al. 2006). However, many individuals without AIP have shown IgG4-related SC with isolated biliary tract involvement (Hamano et al. 2005; Zen et al. 2004). In IgG4-related SC, stenosis is usually observed in the lower part of the common bile duct. The cholangiographic appearance of stenosis in the intrahepatic or hilar hepatic bile duct is very similar to that observed in PSC (Kamisawa and Okamoto 2008), a progressive disease of unknown etiology that ultimately results in liver cirrhosis. IgG4-related SC is associated with older age, male predominance, obstructive jaundice, weight loss, and abdominal discomfort (Kamisawa and Okamoto 2008). Although steroid therapy has shown mixed results in patients with PSC, IgG4-related SC responds dramatically to steroid therapy, as does IgG4RD (Ghazale et al. 2008). The histopathological features of IgG4-related SC are similar to those of AIP and include diffuse plasmacytic infiltration, marked interstitial fibrosis with a focal storiform-like pattern, and obliterative phlebitis.

3.3 *IgG4-Related Dacryoadenitis and Sialoadenitis (Formerly Called Mikulicz's Disease)*

Mikulicz's disease, which is characterized by symmetrical swelling of the lacrimal and salivary glands, is now considered as IgG4-related dacryoadenitis and sialoadenitis in a representative part of the IgG4-RD spectrum (Stone et al. 2012). Different from other organs in IgG4-RD, patients show no gender differences (Yamamoto et al. 2015).

IgG4-related sialadenitis, once considered to be a subset of Sjögren's syndrome (SS), consists of IgG4-related parotitis and IgG4-related submandibular gland disease for salivary glands (parotid and submandibular glands) (Stone et al. 2012). Similar to Mikulicz' disease, Küttner tumor, which refers to enlargement of the unilateral submandibular gland usually associated with IgG4-RD, (Küttner 1896) is replaced by the IgG4-related submandibular gland disease. A clinical comparison of patients with IgG4-RD and those with typical SS shows the following(Umehara et al. 2012): (1) Compared with SS patients, fewer patients with IgG4-RD have symptoms of xerophthalmia, xerostomia, or arthralgia, whereas many have coexisting AIP, interstitial nephritis, allergic rhinitis, and/or bronchial asthma; (2) most patients with IgG4-RD are negative for anti-SS-A and anti-SS-B antibodies, as well as for rheumatoid factor (RF) and anti-nuclear antibody (ANA); (3) serum IgG4 and

IgE concentrations are significantly higher in IgG4-RD than in SS patients; and (4) steroid therapy is extremely effective in patients with IgG4-RD but had limited effect in patients with SS. The most important difference between IgG4-RD and SS is that the former is characterized by marked infiltration of IgG4-positive plasma cells, with a ratio of IgG4-positive to IgG-positive cells of >40 %, a finding almost never seen in patients with SS. Thus, despite their similarities in organ involvement, IgG4-MD and SS are quite different conditions, with distinct clinical and pathological characteristics.

3.4 IgG4-Related Ophthalmic Diseases (IgG4-Related OD)

IgG4-related ophthalmic disease involves not only the lacrimal glands but also other ocular adnexa such as the extraocular muscles and orbital nerves. IgG4-related ophthalmic contains IgG4-related orbital inflammation disease (orbital inflammatory pseudotumor) for orbital soft tissue (or IgG4-related orbital inflammatory pseudotumor), IgG4-related orbital myositis for extraocular muscle disease, and IgG4-related pan-orbital inflammation for orbit with involvement of multiple anatomic structures (Stone et al. 2012). Since the most prominent pathological feature in IgG4-related OD is lymphoplasmacytic cell infiltration, the differential diagnosis is important against MALT lymphoma (extranodal marginal zone B-cell lymphoma of mucosa-associated lymphoid tissue), diffuse large B-cell lymphomas (DLBCL), and follicular lymphoma (Goto et al. 2015).

3.5 IgG4-Related Kidney Disease (IgG4-Related KD)

Mainly tubulointerstitial nephritis (TIN), but occasionally membranous glomerulonephritis (MGN), is observed in IgG4-KD, which shows abundant infiltration of lymphocytes and IgG4-positive plasmacytes, as well as fibrosis (Uchiyama-Tanaka et al. 2004; Takeda et al. 2004). The clinicopathological features of patients with TIN and/or MGN in IgG4-KD usually show proteinuria and/or microhematuria, high serum concentrations of IgG4 and IgE, and hypocomplemententemia, which are somewhat different from other organ lesions in IgG4-RD. IgG4-KD include other conditions than renal parenchymal lesions, such as hydronephrosis due to RPF and tumors of the renal pelvis and urethra. Imaging often shows heterogeneous shadows in the kidneys, such as a mass or multiple nodules that are not observed in other types of interstitial or membranous nephritis.

3.6 IgG4-Related Retroperitoneal Fibrosis (IgG4-Related RPF)

RPF is a chronic fibroinflammatory condition in retroperitoneal tissues. In advanced RPF, involvement of abdominal aorta and hydronephrosis due to obstruction of the ureters is often observed. Although infection, radiation, drugs, malignant tumor, and trauma may be causes of RPF, etiologic factors in many cases are unknown. Histopathological findings are similar to those in AIP or IgG4-related SC, including fibrosis, dense inflammatory cell infiltration with plasma cells and lymphocytes, venulitis, obliterative arteritis, and steroid responsiveness (Neild et al. 2006), which suggests to be categorized as IgG4-RD.

3.7 IgG4-Related Pulmonary Diseases (IgG4-Related PD)

IgG4-related PD shows a great variety of clinical features, which have been described as inflammatory pseudotumor, interstitial pneumonitis, organizing pneumonia, and lymphomatoid granulomatosis (Zen et al. 2009). Although some patients have initially with respiratory symptoms, such as dry cough or dyspnea, about 75 % of patients are asymptomatic and incidentally identified by abnormal shadows on chest X-rays. Although the patients with IgG4-related PD show a variety of radiologic abnormalities (Inoue et al. 2009), diffuse lymphoplasmacytic infiltration is observed in most cases, with irregular fibrosis and obliterative phlebitis being more common in solid areas (Inoue et al. 2009). Radiographically, IgG4-related PD can be divided into two types, inflammatory pseudotumors and interstitial pneumonitis. Inflammatory pseudotumors have been described as nodular or mass lesions, or infiltration, and are characterized by radiating reticular shadows surrounding the tumor. Interstitial pneumonitis presents in most patients with reticular shadows, ground-glass opacity, and interstitial fibrosis in both lower lung fields (Zen et al. 2005). Histopathologically, inflammatory pseudotumor is a plasma cell granuloma, with infiltration mainly by plasma cells and lymphocytes, irregular fibrosis, lymphoid follicle formation, findings of interstitial pneumonitis at the periphery of the nodule, obliterating phlebitis and arteritis, and eosinophilic infiltration (Zen et al. 2005). Interstitial pneumonitis is characterized by thickening of the alveolar septa due to infiltration by plasma cells and lymphocytes, and by diffuse fibrosis.

3.8 IgG4-Related Thyroid Disease

Riedel's thyroiditis was first described in 1896 in two patients with hard goiter and tracheal compressive symptoms (Riedel 1896). One-third of patients with Riedel's thyroiditis have multifocal fibrosclerosis, including sclerosing cholangitis, salivary gland fibrosis, RPF, or fibrotic orbital pseudotumor, which suggests that certain proportions of Riedel's thyroiditis were considered a type of IgG4RD. Different from Riedel's thyroiditis, chronic thyroiditis, the so-called Hashimoto's thyroiditis, has been considered a well-defined clinicopathological entity, characterized by the presence of goiter and serum thyroid autoantibodies. Recently, different from the conventional type of chronic thyroiditis, a unique subtype characterized by the presence of storiform fibrosis, numerous IgG4-positive plasma cells, and elevated serum IgG4 (Li et al. 2009) has been described. Although there were no significant differences in the presence of anti-thyroid and microsome autoantibody between non-IgG4 and IgG4-related thyroid diseases, 60 % of patients with chronic thyroiditis who underwent total thyroidectomy were IgG4-RD (Kakudo et al. 2011).

3.9 IgG4-Related Aortitis/Periaortitis

Aortitis involving the media and periaortitis involving the adventitia and periaortic tissue involving the media sometimes develop to inflammatory aneurysms and dissections. About 40 % of inflammatory abdominal aortic aneurysms (AAAs) are IgG4RD, with elevated IgG4 in serum and abundant infiltration of IgG4 + plasma cells and obliterative phlebitis (Kasashima et al. 2008). IgG4-related periaortitis may exhibit some overlap with IgG4-related retroperitoneal fibrosis.

3.10 IgG4-Related Lymphadenopathy

Lymphadenopathy is often observed in patients with IgG4RD. IgG4-related lymphadenopathy is occasionally characterized by systemic lymphadenopathy, polyclonal hyperimmunoglobulinemia, especially elevated serum levels of IgG, IgG4, and IgE, and the presence of autoantibodies (Umehara et al. 2012; Stone et al. 2012). The IgG4-RD patients with systemic lymphadenopathy should be differed from malignant lymphoma, sarcoidosis, multicentric Castleman's disease, and other malignancies. Histopathologically, IgG4-related lymphadenopathy can be classified into five or subtypes. The former classification contains as type 1; Castleman's disease-like morphology, type II; reactive follicular hyperplasia, type III; interfollicular plasmacytosis and immunoblastosis, type IV; progressive transformation of germinal center-like, type V; and inflammatory pseudotumor-like morphology (Sato et al. 2010). In the latter classification, IgG4-related lymphadenopathy can be divided into two types based on the infiltrative patterns of IgG4-positive cells: interfollicular plasmacytosis (types I, II, III, and V) and intragerminal center plasmacytosis (type IV). Patients with systemic IgG4-related lymphadenopathy usually show significantly lower C-reactive protein (0.29 vs. 8.71 mg/dl) and interleukin (IL)-6 (8.45 vs. 34.82 pg/ml) concentrations than patients with multicentric Castleman's disease (Sato et al. 2009).

Acknowledgment This study was partially supported by (1) Grant-in-Aid for Scientific Research (C) of the Ministry of Culture and Science of Japan (20590810, 24591020, 12008507), (2) the Research Program on Intractable Diseases, from the Ministry of Labor and Welfare of Japan, and (3) grants-in-aid from the Ministry of Education, Culture, Sports, Science and Technology of Japan, from CREST Japan Science, and Technology Agency.

References

Chari ST, Smyrk TC, Levy MJ, Topazian MD, Takahashi N, Zhang L, et al. (2006) Diagnosis of autoimmune pancreatitis: the Mayo Clinic experience. Clin Gastroenterol Hepatol 4:1010–1016

Chari ST, Kloeppel G, Zhang L, Notohara K, Lerch MM, Shimosegawa T et al (2010) Histopathologic and clinical subtypes of autoimmune pancreatitis: the Honolulu consensus document. Pancreas 39:549–554

Cheuk W, Chan AC, Lam WL, Chow SM, Crowley P, Lloydd R et al (2009) IgG4-related sclerosing mastitis: description of a new member of the IgG4-related sclerosing diseases. Am J Surg Pathol 33:1058–1064

Comings DE, Skubi KB, Van Eyes J, Motulsky AG (1967) Familial multifocal fibrosclerosis. Ann Intern Med 66:884–892

Deshpande V, Zen Y, Chan JK, Yi EE, Sato Y, Yoshino T et al (2012) Consensus statement on the pathology of IgG4-related disease. Mod Pathol 25:1181–1192

Ghazale A, Chari ST, Zhang L, Smyrk TC, Takahashi N, Levy MJ et al (2008) Immunoglobulin G4-associated cholangitis: clinical profile and response to therapy. Gastroenterology 134:706–715

Goto H, Takahira M, Azumi A (2015) Japanese study group for IgG4-related ophtalmic disease. Diagnostic criteria for IgG4-related ophthalmic disease. Jpn J Ophthalmol 59:1–7, 2015

Hamano H, Kawa S, Horiuchi A, Unno H, Furuya N, Akamatsu T et al (2001) High serum IgG4 concentrations in patients with sclerosing pancreatitis. N Engl J Med 344:732–738

Hamano H, Kawa S, Ochi Y, Unno H, Shiba N, Wajiki M et al (2002) Hydronephrosis associated with retroperitoneal fibrosis and sclerosing pancreatitis. Lancet 359:1403–1404

Hamano H, Kawa S, Uehara T, Ochi Y, Takayama M, Komatsu K et al (2005) Immunoglobulin G4-related lymphoplasmacytic sclerosing cholangitis that mimics infiltrating hilar cholangiocarcinoma: part of a spectrum of autoimmune pancreatitis? Gastrointest Endosc 62:152–157

Hamano H, Arakura N, Muraki T, Ozaki Y, Kiyosawa K, Kawa S (2006) Prevalence and distribution of extrapancreatic lesions complicating autoimmune pancreatitis. J Gastroenterol 41:1197–1205

Inoue D, Zen Y, Abo H, Gabata T, Demachi H, Kobayashi T et al (2009) Immunoglobulin G4-related lung disease: CT findings with pathologic correlations. Radiology 251:260–270

Japan Pancreas Society (2002) Clinical diagnostic criteria for autoimmune pancreatitis. Suizou 17:585–587

Kakudo K, Li Y, Hirokawa M, Ozaki T (2011) Diagnosis of Hashimoto's thyroiditis and IgG4-related sclerosing disease. Pathol Int 61:175–183

Kamisawa T, Okamoto A (2006) Autoimmune pancreatitis: proposal of IgG4-related sclerosing disease. J Gastroenterol 41:613–625

Kamisawa T, Okamoto A (2008) IgG4-related sclerosing disease. World J Gastroenterol 14:3948–3955

Kamisawa T, Funata N, Hayashi Y, Tsuruta K, Okamoto A, Amemiya K et al (2003) Close relationship between autoimmune pancreatitis and multifocal fibrosclerosis. Gut 52:683–687
Kasashima S, Zen Y, Kawashima A, Konishi K, Sasaki H, Endo M et al (2008) Inflammatory abdominal aortic aneurysm: lose relationship to IgG4-related periaortitis. Am J Surg Pathol 32:197–204
Kawaguchi K, Koike M, Tsuruta K, Okamoto A, Tabata I (1991) Fujita N. Lymphoplasmacytic sclerosing pancreatitis with cholangitis: a variant of primary sclerosing cholangitis extensively involving pancreas. Hum Pathol 22:387–395
Kishimoto M, Okimura Y, Kimura K et al (2000) Multifocal fibrosclerosis as a possible cause of panhypopituitarism with central diabetes insipidus. Endocr J 47:335–342
Klöppel G, Detlefsen S, Chari ST, Longnecker DS, Zamboni G (2010) Autoimmune pancreatitis: the clinicopathological characteristics of the subtype with granulocytic epithelial lesions. J Gastroenterol 45:787–793
Komatsu K, Hamano H, Ochi Y, Takayama M, Muraki T, Yoshizawa K et al (2005) High prevalence of hypothyroidism in patients with autoimmune pancreatitis. Dig Dis Sci 50:1052–1057
Küttner H (1896) U¨ ber entzündiche Tumoren der submaaxilla¨ren Speicheldrüse. Beitr Klin Chir 15:815–834
Küttner K. (1972) Light microscopic determination of nuclear inclusion bodies in juvenilenasopharyngeal fibroma. Z Laryngol Rhinol Otol 51:57–60
Li Y, Bai Y, Liu Z, Ozaki T, Taniguchi E, Mori I et al (2009) Immunohistochemistry of IgG4 can help subclassify Hashimoto's autoimmune thyroiditis. Pathol Int 59:636–641
Li Y, Nishihara E, Hirokawa M, Taniguchi E, Miyauchi A, Kakudo K (2010) Distinct clinical, serological, and sonographic characteristics of hashimoto's thyroiditis based with and without IgG4-positive plasma cells. J Clin Endocrinol Metab 95:1309–1317
Lopes J et al (2010) Autoimmune esophagitis: IgG4-related tumors of the esophagus. J Gastrointest Surg 14:1031–1034
Masaki Y, Dong L, Kurose N, Kitagawa K, Morikawa Y, Yamamoto M et al (2009) Proposal for a new clinical entity, IgG4-positive multi-organ lymphoproliferative syndrome: analysis of 64 cases of IgG4-related disorders. Ann Rheum Dis 68:1310–1315
Matsui S, Taki H, Shinoda K, Suzuki K, Hayashi R, Tobe K et al (2012) Respiratory involvement in IgG4-related Mikulicz's disease. Mod Rheumatol 22:31–39
Mikulicz J (1892) Über eine eigenartige symmetrishe Erkrankung der Tränen und Mundspeicheldrüsen. Beitr z Chir Fesrschr f Theodor Billroth, Stuttgart, pp 610–630
Nakazawa T, Ohara H, Yamada T, Ando H, Sano H, Kajino S et al (2001) Atypical primary sclerosing cholangitis cases associated with unusual pancreatitis. Hepatogastroenterology 48:625–630
Neild GH, Rodriguez-Justo M, Wall C, Connolly JO (2006) Hyper-IgG4 disease: report and characterisation of a new disease. BMC Med 4:23
Nishimori I, Kohsaki T, Onishi S, Shuin T, Kohsaki S, Ogawa Y et al (2007) IgG4-related autoimmune prostatitis: two cases with or without autoimmune pancreatitis. Intern Med 46:1983–1989
Notohara K, Burgart LJ, Yadav D, Chari S, Smyrk TC (2003) Idiopathic chronic pancreatitis with periductal lymphoplasmacytic infiltration: clinicopathologic features of 35 cases. Am J Surg Pathol 27:1119–1127
Okazaki K, Kawa S, Kamisawa T, Naruse S, Tanaka S, Nishimori I, et al. (2006) Research Committee of Intractable Diseases of the Pancreas. Clinical diagnostic criteria of autoimmune pancreatitis: revised proposal. J Gastroenterol. 41:626–631
Okazaki K, Kawa S, Kamisawa T, Ito T, Inui K, Irie H et al (2009) Japanese clinical guidelines for autoimmune pancreatitis. Pancreas 38:849–866
Okazaki K, Uchida K, Koyabu M, Miyoshi H, Takaoka M (2011) Recent advances in the concept and diagnosis of autoimmune pancreatitis and IgG4-related disease. J Gastroenterol 46:277–288
Ravi K, Chari ST, Vege SS, Sandborn WJ, Smyrk TC, Loftus EV Jr (2009) Inflammatory bowel disease in the setting of autoimmune pancreatitis. Inflamm Bowel Dis 15:1326–1330

Riedel BMCL (1896) Die chronische, zur Bildung eisenharter Tumoren fuhrende Entzundung der Schilddruse. Verhandlung der deutsche Gesellschaft furChirurgie 25:101–105

Saegusa H, Momose M, Kawa S, Hamano H, Ochi Y, Takayama M et al (2003) Hilar and pancreatic gallium-67 accumulation is characteristic feature of autoimmune pancreatitis. Pancreas 27:20–25

Sarles H, Sarles JC, Muratore R (1961) Guien C. Chronic inflammatory sclerosis of the pancreas—an autonomous pancreatic disease? Am J Dig Dis 6:688–698

Sato Y, Kojima M, Takata K, Morito T, Asaoku H, Takeuchi T et al (2009) Systemic IgG4-related lymphadenopathy: a clinical and pathologic comparison to multicentric Castleman's disease. Mod Pathol 22:589–599

Sato Y, Notohara K, Kojima M, Takata K, Masaki Y, Yoshino T (2010) IgG4-related disease: historical overview and pathology of hematological disorders. Pathol Int 60:247–258

Sato Y, Takeuchi M, Takata K, Ohno K, Iwaki N, Orita Y, Goto N et al (2012) Clinicopathologic analysis of IgG4-related skin disease. Mod Pathol. doi:10.1038/modpathol.2012

Shimatsu A, Oki Y, Fujiswa I, Sano T (2009) Pituitary and stalk lesions (Infundibulo-hypophysitis) associated with immunoglobulin G4-related systemic disease: an emerging clinical entity. Endocr J 56:1033–1041

Shimosegawa T, Chari ST, Frulloni L, Kamisawa T, Kawa S, Mino-Kenudson M et al (2011) International consensus diagnostic criteria for autoimmune pancreatitis: guidelines of the international association of pancreatology. Pancreas 40:352–358

Stone JH, Khosroshahi A, Hilgenberg A, Spooner A (2009) IsselbacherEM, Stone JR. IgG4-related systemic disease and lymphoplasmacytic aortitis. Arthritis Rheum 60 (10):3139–3145

Stone JH, Khosroshahi A, Deshpande V, Chan JK, Heathcote JG, Aalberse R et al (2012) Recommendations for the nomenclature of IgG4-related disease and its individual organ system manifestations. Arthritis Rheum 64:3061–3067

Takeda S, Haratake J, Kasai T, Takaeda C, Takazakura E (2004) IgG4-associated idiopathic tubulointerstitial nephritis complicating autoimmune pancreatitis. Nephrol Dial Transplant 19:474–476

Uchiyama-Tanaka Y, Mori Y, Kimura T, Watanabe S, Nozaki Y, Fujita K et al (2004) Acute tubulointerstitial nephritis associated with autoimmune-related pancreatitis. Am J Kidney Dis 43:e18–e25

Uehara T, Hamano H, Kawa S, Sano K, Oki K, Kobayashi Y et al (2010) Chronic gastritis in the setting of autoimmune pancreatitis. Am J Surg Pathol 34:1241–1249

Ueno K, Watanabe T, Kawata Y, Gotoh T, Tsuji Y, Ida H et al (2008) IgG4-related autoimmune pancreatitis involving the colonic mucosa. Eur J Gastroenterol Hepatol 20:1118–1121

Umehara H, Okazaki K, Masaki Y, Kawano M, Yamamoto M, Saeki T et al (2012a) A novel clinical entity, IgG4-related disease (IgG4RD): general concept and details. Mod Rheumatol 22:1–14

Umehara H, Okazaki K, Masaki Y, Kawano M, Yamamoto M, Saeki T et al (2012b) Comprehensive diagnostic criteria for IgG4-related disease (IgG4-RD), 2011. Mod Rheumatol 22:21–30

Umemura T, Zen Y, Hamano H, Kawa S, Nakanuma Y, Kiyosawa K (2007) Immunoglobin G4-hepatopathy: association of immunoglobin G4-bearing plasma cells in liver with autoimmune pancreatitis. Hepatology 46:463–471

Umemura T, Zen Y, Hamano H, Joshita S, Ichijo T, Yoshizawa K et al (2011) Clinical significance of immunoglobulin G4-associated autoimmune hepatitis. J Gastroenterol 46(Suppl 1):48–55

Yamamoto M, Takahashi H, Ohara M, Suzuki C, Naishiro Y, Yamamoto H, Shinomura Y, Imai K (2006) A new conceptualization for Mikulicz's disease as an IgG4-related plasmacytic disease. Mod Rheumatol 16:335–340

Yamamoto M, Yajima H, Takahashi H, Yokoyama Y, Ishigami K, Shimizu Y et al (2015) Everyday clinical practice in IgG4-related dacryoadenitis and/or sialadenitis: results from the SMART database. Mod Rheumatol 25:199–204

Yoshida K, Toki F, Takeuchi T, Watanabe S, Shiratori K (1995) Hayashi N. Chronic pancreatitis caused by an autoimmune abnormality. Proposal of the concept of autoimmune pancreatitis. Dig Dis Sci 40:1561–1568

Yoshimura Y, Takeda S, Ieki Y, Takazakura E, Koizumi H, Takagawa K (2006) IgG4-associated prostatitis complicating autoimmune pancreatitis. Intern Med 45:897–901

Zamboni G, Luttges J, Capelli P, Frulloni L, Cavallini G, Pederzoli P et al (2004) Histopathological features of diagnostic and clinical relevance in autoimmune pancreatitis: a study on 53 resection specimens and 9 biopsy specimens. Virchows Arch 445:552–563

Zen Y, Harada K, Sasaki M, Sato Y, Tsuneyama K, Haratake J et al (2004) IgG4-related sclerosing cholangitis with and without hepatic inflammatory pseudotumor, and sclerosing pancreatitis-associated sclerosing cholangitis: do they belong to a spectrum of sclerosing pancreatitis? Am J Surg Pathol 28:1193–1203

Zen Y, Kitagawa S, Minato H, Kuramaya H, Katayanagi K, Masuda S et al (2005) IgG4-positive plasma cells in inflammatory pseudotumor (plasma cell granuloma) of the lung. Hum Pathol 36:710–717

Zen Y, Inoue D, Kitao A, Onodera M, Abo H, Miyayama S et al (2009) IgG4-related lung and pleural disease: a clinicopathologic study of 21 cases. Am J Surg Pathol 33:1886–1893

Diagnosis and Treatment of IgG4-Related Disease

Terumi Kamisawa and Kazuichi Okazaki

Abstract It is critical to differentiate IgG4-related disease (IgG4-RD) from malignant tumor and similar disease of the affected organ to apply appropriate therapy and avoid unnecessary surgery. IgG4-RD is diagnosed on combination of typical radiological findings; elevation of serum IgG4 levels; histopathological findings of abundant infiltration of IgG4-positive plasma cells and lymphocytes, storiform fibrosis, and obliterative phlebitis; association with other IgG4-related diseases; and response to steroids. Histopathological approach is particularly recommended. Systemic glucocorticoids are currently the first-line approach for IgG4-RD, and the indications are symptoms. The initial recommended dose of oral prednisolone for induction of remission is 0.6 mg/kg/day, administered for 2–4 weeks. This dose is gradually tapered to a maintenance dose of 2.5–5 mg/day over a period of 2–3 months. As IgG4-RD sometimes relapses after steroids, maintenance therapy is usually performed in Japan. However, as IgG4-RD patients are typically elderly and are at high risk of developing steroid-related complications, cessation of the medication should be attempted at least within 3 years. For relapsed IgG4-RD, re-administration or dose up of steroid is effective, but the addition of immunomodulatory drugs such as azathioprine has been considered to be appropriate. B cell depletion with rituximab (an anti-CD20 antibody) is effective, even in many patients in whom treatment with immunomodulatory drugs was unsuccessful. The short-term clinical, morphological, and functional outcomes of most IgG4-RD patients treated with steroid therapy are good, but the long-term outcomes are less clear due to several unknown factors such as relapse, developed fibrosis, and associated malignancy.

T. Kamisawa (✉)
Department of Internal Medicine, Tokyo Metropolitan Komagome Hospital,
3-18-22 Honkomagome, Bunkyo-Ku, Tokyo 113-8677, Japan
e-mail: kamisawa@cick.jp

K. Okazaki
Department of Gastroenterology and Hepatology, Kansai Medical University,
Osaka, Japan

Current Topics in Microbiology and Immunology (2017) 401: 19–34
DOI 10.1007/82_2016_36

Published Online: 13 February 2017

Contents

1 Introduction

IgG4-related disease (IgG4-RD) is a recently recognized inflammatory and fibrosing disease of unknown etiology, which can affect almost any organ and is characterized by abundant infiltration of IgG4-positive plasma cells and elevated serum IgG4 levels (Kamisawa et al. 2015). Prior to our proposal of the concept of IgG4-related systemic disease in 2003 (Kamisawa et al. 2003a), manifestations of IgG4-RD were regarded as isolated, organ-specific conditions that included Mikulicz's disease (IgG4-related dacryoadenitis and sialoadenitis), mass-forming pancreatitis [autoimmune pancreatitis (AIP)], Ormond's disease (IgG4-related retroperitoneal fibrosis), and idiopathic pseudotumor (IgG4-related pseudotumor). Some cases of IgG4-RD were surgically resected under the diagnosis of malignancy. While IgG4-RD responds well to steroid treatment, some cases of IgG4-RD relapse after such treatment. In this chapter, we focus on a description of the current status of diagnosis and treatment of IgG4-RD.

2 Diagnosis

Diagnosis of IgG4-RD remains a significant clinical challenge, and there is no simple diagnostic test for IgG4-RD. One problem in diagnosis is that IgG4-RD frequently presents both clinically and radiologically with findings that mimic malignancy. It is therefore critical to differentiate IgG4-RD from malignant tumor of the affected organ (cancer or lymphoma) in an accurate and timely manner to avoid misdiagnosis of malignancy and apply appropriate therapy. It is also recommended to use a histopathological approach to differentiate IgG4-RD from similar diseases of the affected organ [e.g., Sjögren's disease or primary sclerosing cholangitis (PSC)] that can be diagnosed using specific criteria.

2.1 *Epidemiology*

The epidemiology of IgG4-RD is difficult to ascertain. This is because awareness of this disease is low, its diagnosis is sometimes difficult, and its symptoms vary. However, it appears that IgG4-RD is a relatively rare disease. The annual incidence rate of AIP patients was estimated as 1.4 per 100,000 people in Japan in 2011 (Kanno et al. 2015). The incidence of IgG4-RD throughout Japan was estimated as 0.28–1.08/100,000 people, with 336–1300 patients newly diagnosed per year (Umehara et al. 2012a).

In terms of gender distribution, IgG4-RD occurs predominantly in elderly males, and the male-to-female ratio was 3.2 (Kanno et al. 2015). Exceptions are patients with IgG4-related dacryoadenitis and sialadenitis, in whom the gender distribution is almost equal. The mean age of AIP patients was reported as 66.3 years (Kanno et al. 2015).

2.2 *Clinical Symptoms*

The course of IgG4-RD is varied. Some cases improve spontaneously, and the natural course of IgG4-RD is unknown (Kamisawa et al. 2014a). Other cases of IgG4-RD may have a subacute or a chronic course. The clinical symptoms of IgG4-RD also vary and depend on the pattern of organ involvement and the severity of the disease activity. Thus, although severe constitutional symptoms are rare, organomegaly or hypertrophy can cause serious complications of obstruction or compression in some patients including obstructive jaundice in AIP or IgG4-related sclerosing cholangitis; visual disturbance in IgG4-related dacryoadenitis; and hydronephrosis in IgG4-related retroperitoneal fibrosis. Furthermore, persistent inflammation in affected organs has been shown to lead to fibrosis and permanent organ dysfunction or failure. Examples of such complications include exocrine and endocrine pancreatic dysfunction in AIP, liver fibrosis in IgG4-related sclerosing cholangitis, and renal dysfunction in IgG4-related kidney disease (Khosroshahi et al. 2015).

In addition, many patients with IgG4-RD have a history of allergic disease or atopic features (Kamisawa et al. 2009b).

2.3 Laboratory Tests

Although most patients with IgG4-RD have elevated serum IgG4-levels, IgG4RD cannot be diagnosed solely on the basis of serum IgG4 levels for the following reasons. First, even though elevated serum IgG4 levels (to greater than 135 mg/dl) were reported in 84 % (1586/1883) of patients with IgG4-RD, and the mean serum IgG4 level was 769 mg/dl (Stone et al. 2015), some patients with early or limited stage of IgG4-RD do not present with high IgG4 levels. Second, elevation of serum IgG4 levels is not restricted to IgG4-RD and is also seen in other conditions such as autoimmune disease, allergic conditions, carcinoma, and Castleman's disease. Indeed, a recent study reported that elevated serum IgG4 levels by themselves have a low specificity (60 %) and a low positive predictive value (34 %) for the diagnosis of IgG4-RD (Carruthers et al. 2015a). Therefore, if serum IgG4 levels are to be taken into account in the diagnosis of IgG4-RD, then rigorous clinicopathological correlation is required.

Routine laboratory tests often provide nonspecific indications of organ involvement in IgG4-RD that require further examination. For example, 34 % of patients with IgG4-RD were reported to have peripheral eosinophilia (Stone et al. 2015). Polyclonal hypergammaglobulinemia, elevation of IgE, the presence of antinuclear antigen, and the presence of rheumatoid factor were found in 61, 58, 30, and 20 % of IgG4-RD patients, respectively, in serological tests. Hypocomplementemia, which is particularly common in patients with IgG4-related kidney disease, was observed in 41 % of IgG4-RD patients (Stone et al. 2015).

2.4 Imaging

CT scanning, MRI imaging, and 18 F-fluorodeoxyglucose positron emission tomography/computed tomography (FDG-PET/CT) are popular methods of imaging IgG4-RD. On enhanced CT images of IgG4-RD, a diffuse or focal swelling of organs or soft tissue masses appears with soft tissue attenuation, well-defined margins, and homogeneous enhancement at late stage. These findings present as iso- to hypointense on T2-weighted MRI and reflect increased cellularity and fibrosis (Fujita et al. 2012). FDG-PET/CT is useful for mapping the sites of IgG4-RD by highlighting hypermetabolic activity (Nakatani et al. 2012).

It is sometimes possible to differentiate IgG4-RD from other diseases on the basis of characteristic imaging features of some organs. For example, AIP may be differentiated from pancreatic cancer based on imaging features. Thus, on CT images, typical AIP shows diffuse enlargement of the pancreas with delayed enhancement in association with a capsule-like low-density rim (Fig. 1). On endoscopic retrograde cholangiopancreatography (ERCP) or magnetic resonance cholangiopancreatography (MRCP), AIP shows diffuse irregular narrowing of the main pancreatic duct (Fig. 2). On pancreatography, AIP rather than pancreatic

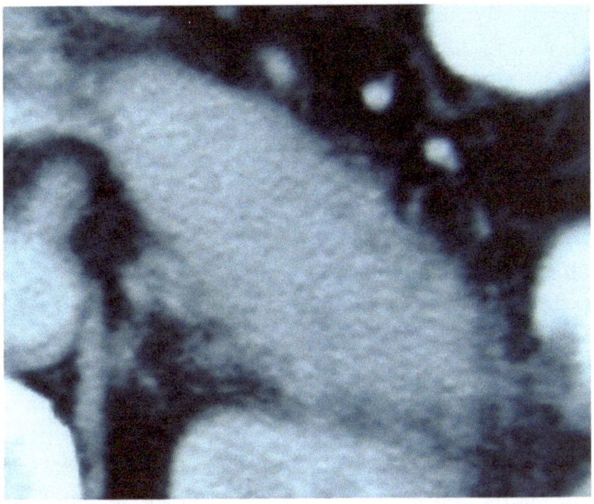

Fig. 1 CT scan in a patient with autoimmune pancreatitis showing enlargement of the pancreatic body and tail with delayed enhancement

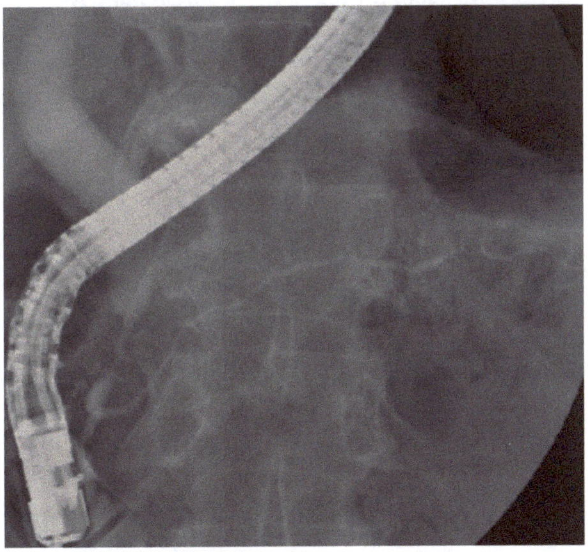

Fig. 2 Endoscopic retrograde cholangiopancreatography in a patient with autoimmune pancreatitis showing diffuse irregular narrowing of the main pancreatic duct and stenosis of the lower bile duct

cancer is suggested by long narrowing of the main pancreatic duct, skipped narrowed lesions, side branch derivation from the narrowed portion, and less upstream dilatation (Kamisawa et al. 2008). In AIP patients, the lower bile duct is frequently stenotic (Fig. 2). Imaging may also help to differentiate IgG4-related sclerosing cholangitis from PSC and hilar cholangiocarcinoma. Thus, dominant cholangiographic findings for PSC that are rarely observed in patients with IgG4-related sclerosing cholangitis include band-like stricture, a beaded or pruned-tree appearance, and diverticulum-like outpouching, while IgG4-related sclerosing cholangitis commonly displays dilatation after a long stricture of the bile duct. While cholangiography cannot distinguish IgG4-related sclerosing cholangitis from hilar cholangiocarcinoma, IgG4-related sclerosing cholangitis rather than cholangiocarcinoma is highly suggested by wall thickness in the bile duct that appears normal in the cholangiogram on endoscopic ultrasonography or intraductal ultrasonography (Ohara et al. 2012; Kamisawa et al. 2014b).

Imaging features that are commonly found in other IgG4-RDs include the following. In IgG4-related sialadenitis, the submandibular glands are more commonly affected than the parotid glands. In IgG4-related dacryoadenitis, in addition to (often bilateral) lacrimal glands, other tissues, such as extraocular muscles, orbital fat tissues, eyelids, trigeminal nerve branches, and nasolacrimal duct, are sometimes involved (Koizumi et al. 2014). In IgG4-related lung disease, common imaging findings are thickening of the perilymphatic interstitium and mediastinal lymphadenopathy with or without subpleural and/or peribronchovascular consolidation (Matsui et al. 2013). In IgG4-related kidney disease, characteristic imaging findings are multiple low-density lesions on enhanced CT, diffuse kidney enlargement, hypovascular solitary mass in the kidney, and hypertrophic lesion of the renal pelvic wall without irregularity of the renal pelvic surface (Kawano et al. 2011). In IgG4-related retroperitoneal fibrosis, a soft tissue mass surrounding the aorta and/or adjacent tissues, sometimes with hydronephrosis, is observed (Chiba et al. 2013).

2.5 Histopathology

The current gold standard for the diagnosis of IgG4-RD is its characteristic histology and immunohistochemistry, which is almost the same regardless of the organs involved. Major histopathological features of IgG4-RD are dense lymphoplasmacytic infiltration with storiform fibrosis, obliterative phlebitis, and abundant infiltration of IgG4-positive plasma cells. However, some of these features can also be found in other diseases. For example, the presence of significant infiltration of IgG4-positive plasma cells in a biopsied specimen is not specific to IgG4-RD. Extensive IgG4-positive plasma cell infiltration has been described in other conditions that commonly mimic IgG4-RD, including malignancy. It is therefore important to differentiate IgG4-RD from malignant tumors of each organ and from similar diseases by additional adequate histopathological examination. One method that may help to distinguish IgG4-RD from other conditions is semiquantitative analysis of immunostaining. A frequently used cutof immunostaining. A frequently used cutoff value of infiltrated IgG4-positive plasma cells is more than 10 cells per high-power field (HPF), but the cutoff value varies according to the specific tissue. Measurement of the IgG4-positive cell/total IgG-positive cell ratio, in which a minimum ratio of 40 % is usually used, may also be useful, especially in cases in which fibrosis is predominant. Although findings of storiform fibrosis and obliterative phlebitis enhance diagnostic specificity, clinicopathological correlation is always essential (Deshpande et al. 2012).

However, a problem with IgG4-RD analysis based on histopathology is that IgG4-RD-related histopathology can vary according to the stage of the disease. Confirmation of a diagnosis of IgG4-RD in long-standing IgG4-RD using histopathology can be difficult, since the tissue may have become predominantly fibrotic. Although malignancies can generally be excluded by needle biopsies, such biopsies often provide insufficient quantities of tissue to allow confirmation of a diagnosis of IgG4-RD. Samples from previous biopsied or resected specimens may be diagnostic if they are reviewed along with IgG4-immunostaining of paraffin-embedded specimens (Khosroshahi et al. 2015).

2.6 *Steroid Responsiveness*

Response to steroids can confirm a strong suspicion of the presence of IgG4-RD in patients with appropriate collateral evidence. In cases in which sufficient biopsy specimens cannot be obtained, such as cases where specimens are obtained from the biliary tract, it is difficult to differentiate IgG4-RD from malignancy, and, in such cases, a steroid trial can be applied. However, such a diagnostic steroid trial should be conducted carefully after a negative workup for malignancy that includes a histopathological approach. Furthermore, a steroid trial should only be applied to cases in which the effect of steroid therapy can be evaluated by imaging modalities, since symptomatic and hematological improvements occur nonspecifically in response to steroids, even in malignancy (Kamisawa et al. 2014a; Shimosegawa et al. 2011).

2.7 *Diagnostic Criteria*

Specific diagnostic criteria have been established for IgG4-RD in each of four organs: AIP (Shimosegawa et al. 2011); IgG4-related sclerosing cholangitis (Ohara et al. 2012); IgG4-related kidney disease (Kawano et al. 2011); and IgG4-related sialadenitis and dacryoadenitis (Mikulicz's disease) (Masaki et al. 2010). These criteria are roughly based on a combination of the following findings: typical radiological findings; elevation of serum IgG4 levels; histopathological findings of abundant infiltration of IgG4-positive plasma cells and lymphocytes, storiform fibrosis, and obliterative phlebitis; association with other IgG4-related diseases; and response to steroids. Comprehensive diagnostic criteria for IgG4-RD that are independent of the predominant organ involvement have been proposed for practical use by general clinicians and non-specialists (Table 1) (Umehara et al. 2012b).

Table 1 Comprehensive diagnostic criteria for IgG4-related disease, 2011

1. Clinical examination showing characteristic diffuse/localized swelling or masses in single or multiple organs	
2. Hematological examination shows elevated serum IgG4 concentrations (≥135 mg/dl)	
3. Histopathological examination shows:	
	(1) Marked lymphocyte and plasmacyte infiltration and fibrosis
	(2) Infiltration of IgG4+plasma cells: ration of IgG4+/IgG +cells > 40 % and > 10 IgG4+plasma cells/HPF
	Definite: 1) + 2) + 3)
	Probable: 1) + 3)
	Possible: 1) + 2)

Minimal criteria proposed to consider a previously unrecognized organ or site as being involved in IgG4-RD are appropriate histopathological findings (such findings are essential), with at least one additional criterion of serology, steroid responsiveness, and other organ involvement (Deshpande et al. 2012).

3 Treatment

Although an international consensus guidance statement on the management and treatment of IgG4-RD was proposed in 2015 (Khosroshahi et al. 2015), no international treatment guidelines exist, and currently the treatment strategy for AIP is somewhat different in Asian and Western countries. In Japan, the Japanese consensus guidelines for treatment of AIP were revised in 2014 (Kamisawa et al. 2014a). Systemic glucocorticoids are currently the first-line approach for IgG4-RD. However, several approaches to the management of AIP have been reported, including systemic steroids, steroid-sparing immunosuppressive drugs, and biological agents. A definitive treatment strategy for IgG-RD remains to be established.

3.1 Indication of Treatment

It is essential that accurate diagnosis of IgG4-RD is confirmed before starting treatment.

Spontaneous improvement is observed in some cases of IgG4-RD (Kamisawa et al. 2014a). Therefore, in asymptomatic patients with focal pancreatic enlargement, mild submandibular gland enlargement, or lymphadenopathy, it may be appropriate to provide conservative follow-up.

However, uncontrolled disease in certain organs can lead to irreversible damage. Urgent treatment is therefore recommended for the following types of IgG4-RD: aortitis, retroperitoneal fibrosis, sclerosing cholangitis, tubulointerstitial nephritis, pachymeningitis, and pericarditis (Khosroshahi et al. 2015). It is generally accepted that indications for steroid therapy in IgG4-RD patients are symptoms. A recent international multicenter study of the long-term outcomes of AIP indicated that jaundice (63 %, 458/724) was the most common indication for steroid therapy in AIP patients (Hart et al. 2013a). Some cases of markedly fibrotic or advanced diseases (so-called burned-out cases) may show a poor response to steroids (Shimizu et al. 2013).

3.2 Induction of Remission

The first goal of therapy in IgG4-RD is to induce remission. Glucocorticoids are the first-line agent for remission induction in all patients with acute, untreated IgG4-RD unless contraindications to such treatment are present. Glucocorticoids are used since response to steroid therapy in IgG4-RD patients is dramatic and consistently leads to clinical improvement.

For treatment of AIP, the Japanese guidelines (Kamisawa et al. 2014a) indicate that, before steroid therapy, obstructive jaundice should be controlled by biliary drainage, and blood glucose levels should be controlled in patients with diabetes mellitus, generally by using insulin. The initial recommended dose of oral prednisolone for induction of remission is 0.6 mg/kg/day, administered for 2–4 weeks. This dose is gradually tapered to a maintenance dose of 2.5–5 mg/day over a period of 2–3 months (Fig. 3). Steroid pulse therapy has been reported to be useful and may prevent unnecessary surgery when oral steroid therapy is not indicated because of the required period for drug tapering (Matsushita et al. 2007).

Response to steroids is assessed by periodic biochemical and serological blood tests, such as tests of liver enzymes and IgG4 levels, respectively, as well as by imaging tests, such as CT, MRCP, and ERCP. Pancreatic size usually normalizes within a few weeks, and biliary drainage becomes unnecessary within about 1 month. A rapid response to steroids confirms the diagnosis of AIP and IgG4-SC.

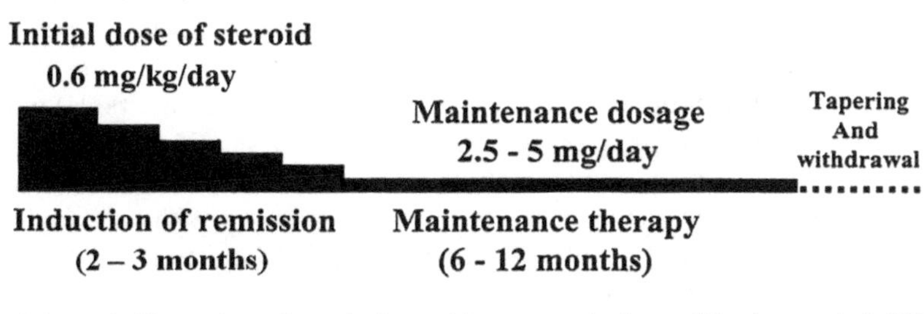

Fig. 3 Schematic illustration of standard steroid treatment in Japan (Kamisawa et al. 2014a, b)

However, if steroid effectiveness is reduced, the patient should be re-evaluated for suspected pancreatic cancer (Kamisawa et al. 2014a).

3.3 Relapse and Maintenance Therapy

Relapse of IgG4-RD is defined as the reappearance of symptoms with the reappearance of imaging abnormalities, and/or elevation of serum IgG4 levels.

In a Japanese multicenter survey of AIP (Kamisawa et al. 2009a), steroid therapy significantly lowered the relapse rate of AIP, with the relapse rate being 24 % (110/451) in those who received steroid therapy compared to 42 % (32/77; $p < 0.01$) in those not given steroid therapy. In the patients who received steroid therapy, relapse occurred in the pancreas ($n = 57$, 52 %), bile duct ($n = 37$, 34 %), and extrapancreatic lesions.

Whether maintenance steroid therapy benefits AIP patients is still unconfirmed. In a Japanese survey of AIP (Kamisawa et al. 2009a), maintenance steroid therapy was given after remission in 377 (82 %) of 459 patients that were treated with steroid. The relapse rate of patients with maintenance therapy was 23 % (63/273), which was significantly lower than that of patients who stopped maintenance therapy (34 %, 35/104; $p < 0.05$). The relapse rate of AIP patients treated with steroid in Korea, where maintenance therapy was stopped completely after about 6 months, was 33 % (13/40) (Park et al. 2008). The reported relapse rates of patients treated with steroid in the USA and the UK, where no maintenance therapy was given, were 38–60 % (Ghazale et al. 2008; Sandanayake et al. 2009; Raina et al. 2009). Given these findings, maintenance therapy with low-dose prednisolone (2.5–5 mg/day) was recommended to prevent relapse.

However, some patients do not relapse without maintenance therapy, and some patients relapse during steroid tapering or during maintenance therapy with relatively high doses of prednisolone. Therefore, it is important to evaluate disease activity in the patient in order to judge the indications of maintenance therapy. Patients at a higher risk of relapse are those with multi-organ disease, significant elevation of serum IgG4 levels, and proximal extrahepatic/intrahepatic biliary strictures, or those with a history of relapse (Kamisawa et al. 2009a, 2014a). These patients with an elevated risk of relapse will likely benefit from maintenance therapy in an effort to minimize morbidity. However, as IgG4-RD patients are typically elderly and are at high risk of developing steroid-related complications such as osteoporosis and diabetes mellitus, cessation of the medication should be attempted. A Japanese multicenter study of AIP (Kamisawa et al. 2009a) indicated that the cumulative rate of relapse ($n = 99$) after starting steroid therapy was 56 % at 1 year, 76 % at 2 years, and 92 % after 3 years. Cessation of maintenance therapy should be planned within at least 3 years in cases with radiological and serological improvement. It is necessary to evaluate disease activity when stopping medication, and after stopping medication, patients should be followed up for relapse.

For relapsed AIP, re-administration or dose up of steroid was shown to be effective.

In cases where the steroid dosage cannot be tapered due to persistently active disease, the addition of immunomodulatory drugs such as azathioprine, mycophenolate mofetil, or 6-mercaptopurine has been considered to be appropriate (Ghazale et al. 2008; Sandanayake et al. 2009; Raina et al. 2009). However, in a retrospective study that compared treatment of patients who had relapsing AIP with immunomodulatory drugs to steroid monotherapy, no significant difference in relapse-free survival was observed between the 2 groups (Hart et al. 2013b).

Retrospective studies suggest that B cell depletion with rituximab (an anti-CD20 antibody) is effective, even in many patients in whom treatment with immunomodulatory drugs was unsuccessful (Topazian et al. 2008; Khosroshahi et al. 2012). A recent prospective study reported that disease response was observed in 97 % of patients with IgG4-related disease who were treated with rituximab (Carruthers et al. 2015a,b). The effect of rituximab has been attributed, at least in part, to a failure of repletion of short-lived plasma blasts or plasma cells that produce IgG4 in IgG4-RD (Kamisawa et al. 2015).

3.4 Treatment–Related Side Effects

Treatment-related side effects were reported in a Japanese study of 459 AIP patients treated with steroid (Kamisawa et al. 2009a). These effects included mildly or moderately worse glucose tolerance in several patients; osteoporosis, including compression fractures of lumbar vertebrae ($n = 5$) and avascular necrosis of the femoral head ($n = 3$), in 10 patients; and pneumonia in 3 patients. However, these effects could be controlled with medical treatment and reduction in dosage or cessation of medication.

Side effects of immunosuppressive drugs were reported in a study by the Mayo Clinic (Hart et al. 2013b). In that study, nine (22 %) of 41 patients treated with immunosuppressive drugs required drug discontinuation (azathioprine or 6-mercaptopurine) for nausea/vomiting ($n = 4$), transaminitis ($n = 2$), bacteremia ($n = 1$), drug rash ($n = 1$), or myelosuppression ($n = 1$). Side effects seen in three (25 %) of 12 patients treated with rituximab included infusion reaction (chills and headache, $n = 1$), late-onset neutropenia, and probable bronchiolitis obliterans organizing pneumonia.

4 Prognosis

The short-term clinical, morphological, and functional outcomes of most IgG4-RD patients treated with steroid therapy are good, although the long-term outcomes are less clear. Thus, after steroid therapy, pancreatic endocrine and exocrine functions improve in half of AIP patients, and salivary and lacrimal gland function improve in patients with IgG4-related sialadenitis and dacryoadenitis (Kamisawa et al. 2003a, b). However, there are several unknown factors such as relapse, developed fibrosis, and associated malignancy that influence long-term outcomes. For example, pancreatic stones form in relapsing AIP patients, which might be induced by pancreatic juice stasis from intensified incomplete obstruction of the pancreatic duct system (Hart et al. 2013a, b; Kamisawa et al. 2014a, b).

It has also been reported that the risk of malignancy is high in patients with IgG4-RD (Yamamoto et al. 2012). There are a few reports of an AIP case developing pancreatic cancer, but it is unclear whether there is a relationship between AIP and pancreatic cancer (Kamisawa et al. 2014a). However, as IgG4-RD occurs predominantly in elderly males and steroid therapy is immunosuppressive, imaging and serum tumor markers should be periodically checked during follow-up.

5 Future Perspectives

Early detection of IgG4-RD requires greater awareness of this disease in the medical community. Furthermore, it is necessary to identify more reliable biomarkers than serum IgG4 levels for the assessment of longitudinal disease activity.

With respect to the initial management of IgG4-RD, there is still no consensus regarding the details of the steroid regimen to be used to induce remission, including the duration of induction therapy and the tapering schedule, and it is still unknown which patients might benefit from maintenance therapy. Additionally, the choice of medication (steroid, immunosuppressive drugs, or rituximab) and the optimal duration of maintenance therapy need to be standardized. These points need to be addressed in international, randomized, controlled clinical trials.

References

Carruthers MN, Khosroshahi A, Augustin T, Deshpande V, Stone JH (2015a) The diagnostic utility of serum IgG4 concentrations in IgG4-related disease. Ann Rheum Dis 74(1):14–18. doi:10.1136/annrheumdis-2013-204907

Carruthers MN, Topazian MD, Khosroshahi A, Witzig TE, Wallace ZS, Hart PA, Deshpande V, Smyrk TC, Chari S, Stone JH (2015b) Rituximab for IgG4-related disease: a prospective, open-label trial. Ann Rheum Dis 74(6):1171–1177. doi:10.1136/annrheumdis-2014-206605

Chiba K, Kamisawa T, Tabata T, Hara S, Kuruma S, Fujiwara T, Kuwata G, Egashira H, Koizumi K, Koizumi S, Fujiwara J, Arakawa T, Momma K, Setoguchi K, Shinohara M (2013) Clinical features of 10 patients with IgG4-related retroperitoneal fibrosis. Intern Med 52 (14):1545–1551

Deshpande V, Zen Y, Chan JK, Yi EE, Sato Y, Yoshino T, Klöppel G, Heathcote JG, Khosroshahi A, Ferry JA, Aalberse RC, Bloch DB, Brugge WR, Bateman AC, Carruthers MN, Chari ST, Cheuk W, Cornell LD, Fernandez-Del Castillo C, Forcione DG, Hamilos DL,

Kamisawa T, Kasashima S, Kawa S, Kawano M, Lauwers GY, Masaki Y, Nakanuma Y, Notohara K, Okazaki K, Ryu JK, Saeki T, Sahani DV, Smyrk TC, Stone JR, Takahira M, Webster GJ, Yamamoto M, Zamboni G, Umehara H, Stone JH (2012) Consensus statement on the pathology of IgG4-related disease. Mod Pathol 25(9):1181–1192. doi:10.1038/modpathol.2012.72

Fujita A, Sakai O, Chapman MN, Sugimoto H (2012) IgG4-related disease of the head and neck CT and MR imaging manifestations. Radiographics 32(7):1945–1958

Ghazale A, Chari ST, Zhang L, Smyrk TC, Takahashi N, Levy MJ, Topazian MD, Clain JE, Pearson RK, Petersen BT, Vege SS, Lindor K, Farnell MB (2008) Immunoglobulin G4-associated cholangitis: clinical profile and response to therapy. Gastroenterology 134 (3):706–715

Hart PA, Kamisawa T, Brugge WR, Chung JB, Culver EL, Czakó L, Frulloni L, Go VL, Gress TM, Kim MH, Kawa S, Lee KT, Lerch MM, Liao WC, Löhr M, Okazaki K, Ryu JK, Schleinitz N, Shimizu K, Shimosegawa T, Soetikno R, Webster G, Yadav D, Zen Y, Chari ST (2013a) Long-term outcomes of autoimmune pancreatitis: a multicentre, international analysis. Gut 62(12):1771–1776. doi:10.1136/gutjnl-2012-303617

Hart PA, Topazian MD, Witzig TE, Clain JE, Gleeson FC, Klebig RR, Levy MJ, Pearson RK, Petersen BT, Smyrk TC, Sugumar A, Takahashi N, Vege SS, Chari ST (2013b) Treatment of relapsing autoimmune pancreatitis with immunomodulators and rituximab: the Mayo Clinic experience. Gut 62:1607–1615

Kamisawa T, Funata N, Hayashi Y, Eishi Y, Koike M, Tsuruta K, Okamoto A, Egawa N, Nakajima H (2003a) A new clinicopathological entity of IgG4-related autoimmune disease. J Gastroenterol 38(10):982–984

Kamisawa T, Egawa N, Inokuma S, Tsuruta K, Okamoto A, Kamata N, Nakamura T, Matsukawa M (2003b) Pancreatic endocrine and exocrine function and salivary gland function in autoimmune pancreatitis before and after steroid therapy. Pancreas 27(3):235–238

Kamisawa T, Imai M, Yui Chen P, Tu Y, Egawa N, Tsuruta K, Okamoto A, Suzuki M, Kamata N (2008) Strategy for differentiating autoimmune pancreatitis from pancreatic cancer. Pancreas 37(3):e62–e67. doi:10.1097/MPA.0b013e318175e3a0

Kamisawa T, Shimosegawa T, Okazaki K, Nishino T, Watanabe H, Kanno A, Okumura F, Nishikawa T, Kobayashi K, Ichiya T, Takatori H, Yamakita K, Kubota K, Hamano H, Okamura K, Hirano K, Ito T, Ko SB, Omata M (2009a) Standard steroid treatment for autoimmune pancreatitis. Gut 58:1504–1507

Kamisawa T, Anjiki H, Egawa N, Kubota N (2009b) Allergic manifestations in autoimmune pancreatitis. Eur J Gastroenterol Hepatol 21(10):1136–1139

Kamisawa T, Okazaki K, Kawa S, Ito T, Inui K, Irie H, Nishino T, Notohara K, Nishimori I, Tanaka S, Nishiyama T, Suda K, Shiratori K, Tanaka M, Shimosegawa T; Working Committee of the Japan Pancreas Society and the Research Committee for Intractable Pancreatic Disease supported by the Ministry of Health, Labour and Welfare of Japan (2014a) Amendment of the Japanese Consensus Guidelines for Autoimmune Pancreatitis, 2013 III. Treatment and prognosis of autoimmune pancreatitis. J Gastroenterol 49(6):961–70. doi:10.1007/s00535-014-0945-z

Kamisawa T, Ohara H, Kim MH, Kanno A, Okazaki K, Fujita N (2014b) Role of endoscopy in the diagnosis of autoimmune pancreatitis and immunoglobulin G4-related sclerosing cholangitis. Dig Endosc 26(5):627–635. doi:10.1111/den.12289

Kamisawa T, Zen Y, Pillai JH Stone (2015) IgG4-related disease. Lancet 385(9976):1460–1471

Kanno A, Masamune A, Okazaki K, Kamisawa T, Kawa S, Nishimori I, Tsuji I, Shimosegawa T (2015) Nationwide epidemiological survey of autoimmune pancreatitis in Japan in 2011. Pancreas 44(4):535–539

Kawano M, Saeki T, Nakashima H, Nishi S, Yamaguchi Y, Hisano S, Yamanaka N, Inoue D, Yamamoto M, Takahashi H, Nomura H, Taguchi T, Umehara H, Makino H, Saito T (2011) Proposal for diagnostic criteria for IgG4-related kidney disease. Clin Exp Nephrol 15(5):615–626. doi:10.1007/s10157-011-0521-2

Khosroshahi A, Carruthers MN, Deshpande V, Unizony S, Bloch DB, Stone JH (2012) Rituximab for the treatment of IgG4-related disease: lessons from 10 consecutive patients. Medicine (Baltimore) 91(1):57–66. doi:10.1097/MD.0b013e3182431ef6

Khosroshahi A, Wallace ZS, Crowe JL, Akamizu T, Azumi A, Carruthers MN, Chari ST, Della-Torre E, Frulloni L, Goto H, Hart PA, Kamisawa T, Kawa S, Kawano M, Kim MH, Kodama Y, Kubota K, Lerch MM, Löhr M, Masaki Y, Matsui S, Mimori T, Nakamura S, Nakazawa T, Ohara H, Okazaki K, Ryu JH, Saeki T, Schleinitz N, Shimatsu A, Shimosegawa T, Takahashi H, Takahira M, Tanaka A, Topazian M, Umehara H, Webster GJ, Witzig TE, Yamamoto M, Zhang W, Chiba T, Stone JH; Second International Symposium on IgG4-Related Disease (2015) International consensus guidance statement on the management and treatment of IgG4-related disease. Arthritis Rheumatol 67(7):1688–1699. doi:10.1002/art.39132

Koizumi S, Kamisawa T, Kuruma S, Tabata T, Iwasaki S, Chiba K, Setoguchi K, Horiguchi S, Ozaki N (2014) Clinical features of IgG4-related dacryoadenitis. Graefes Arch Clin Exp Ophthalmol 252(3):491–497. doi:10.1007/s00417-013-2541-y

Masaki Y, Sugai S, Umehara H (2010) IgG4-related diseases including Mikulicz's disease and sclerosing pancreatitis: diagnostic insights. J Rheum 37:1380–1385

Matsui S, Hebisawa A, Sakai F, Yamamoto H, Terasaki Y, Kurihara Y, Waseda Y, Kawamura T, Miyashita T, Inoue H, Hata N, Masubuchi H, Sugino K, Kishi J, Kobayashi H, Usui Y, Komazaki Y, Kawabata Y, Ogura T (2013) Immunoglobulin G4-related lung disease: clinicoradiological and pathological features. Respirology 18(3):480–487. doi:10.1111/resp.12016

Matsushita M, Yamashina M, Ikeura T, Shimatani M, Uchida K, Takaoka M, Okazaki K (2007) Effective steroid pulse therapy for the biliary stenosis caused by autoimmune pancreatitis. Am J Gastroenterol 102(1):220–221

Nakatani K, Nakamoto Y, Togashi K (2012) Utility of FDG PET/CT in IgG4-related systemic disease. Clin Radiol 67(4):297–305

Ohara H, Okazaki K, Tsubouchi H, Inui K, Kawa S, Kamisawa T, Tazuma S, Uchida K, Hirano K, Yoshida H, Nishino T, Ko SB, Mizuno N, Hamano H, Kanno A, Notohara K, Hasebe O, Nakazawa T, Nakanuma Y, Takikawa H; Research Committee of IgG4-related Diseases; Research Committee of Intractable Diseases of Liver and Biliary Tract; Ministry of Health, Labor and Welfare, Japan; Japan Biliary Association (2012) Clinical diagnostic criteria of IgG4-related sclerosing cholangitis 2012. J Hepatobiliary Pancreat Sci 19:536–542

Park DH, Kim MH, Oh HB, Kwon OJ, Choi YJ, Lee SS, Lee TY, Seo DW, Lee SK (2008) Substitution of aspartic acid at position 57 of the DQβ1 affects relapse of autoimmune pancreatitis. Gastroenterology 134:440–446

Raina A, Yadav D, Krasinskas AM, McGrath KM, Khalid A, Sanders M, Whitcomb DC, Slivka A (2009) Evaluation and management of autoimmune pancreatitis: experience at a large US center. Am J Gastroenterol 104(9):2295–2306. doi:10.1038/ajg.2009.325

Sandanayake NS, Church NI, Chapman MH, Johnson GJ, Dhar DK, Amin Z, Deheragoda MG, Novelli M, Winstanley A, Rodriguez-Justo M, Hatfield AR, Pereira SP, Webster GJ (2009) Presentation and management of post-treatment relapse in autoimmune pancreatitis/immunoglobulin G4-associated cholangitis. Clin Gastroenterol Hepatol 7(10):1089–1096

Shimosegawa T, Chari ST, Frulloni L, Kamisawa T, Kawa S, Mino-Kenudson M, Kim MH, Kloppel G, Lerch MM, Lohr M, Notohara K, Okazaki K, Schneider A, Zhang L (2011) International consensus diagnostic criteria for autoimmune pancreatitis. Guidelines of the International Association of Pancreatology. Pancreas 40:352–358

Shimizu Y, Yamamoto M, Naishiro Y, Sudoh G, Ishigami K, Yajima H, Tabeya T, Matsui M, Suzuki C, Takahashi H, Seki N, Himi T, Yamashita K, Noguchi H, Hasegawa T, Suzuki Y, Honda S, Abe T, Imai K, Shinomura Y (2013) Necessity of early intervention for IgG4-related disease–delayed treatment induces fibrosis progression. Rheumatology (Oxford) 52:679–683

Stone JH, Brito-Zerón P, Bosch X, Ramos-Casals M (2015) Diagnostic approach to the complexity of IgG4-related disease. Mayo Clin Proc 90(7):927–939. doi:10.1016/j.mayocp.2015.03.020

Topazian M, Witzig TE, Smyrk TC, Pulido JS, Levy MJ, Kamath PS, Chari ST (2008) Rituximab therapy for refractory biliary strictures in immunoglobulin G4-associated cholangitis. Clin Gastroenterol Hepatol 6(3):364–646. doi:10.1016/j.cgh.2007.12.020

Umehara H, Okazaki K, Masaki Y, Kawano M, Yamamoto M, Saeki T, Matsui S, Sumida T, Mimori T, Tanaka Y, Tsubota K, Yoshino T, Kawa S, Suzuki R, Takegami T, Tomosugi N, Kurose N, Ishigaki Y, Azumi A, Kojima M, Nakamura S, Inoue D; Research Program for Intractable Disease by Ministry of Health, Labor and Welfare (MHLW) Japan G4 team (2012a) A novel clinical entity, IgG4-related disease (IgG4RD): general concept and details. Mod Rheumatol 22(1):1–14. doi:10.1007/s10165-011-0508-6

Umehara H, Okazaki K, Masaki Y, Kawano M, Yamamoto M, Saeki T, Matsui S, Yoshino T, Nakamura S, Kawa S, Hamano H, Kamisawa T, Shimosegawa T, Shimatsu A, Nakamura S, Ito T, Notohara K, Sumida T, Tanaka Y, Mimori T, Chiba T, Mishima M, Hibi T, Tsubouchi H, Inui K, Ohara H (2012b) Comprehensive diagnostic criteria for IgG4-related disease (IgG4-RD), 2011. Mod Rheumatol 22:21–30

Yamamoto M, Takahashi H, Tabeya T, Suzuki C, Naishiro Y, Ishigami K, Yajima H, Shimizu Y, Obara M, Yamamoto H, Himi T, Imai K, Shinomura Y (2012) Risk of malignancies in IgG4-related disease. Mod Rheumatol 22(3):414–418. doi:10.1007/s10165-011-0520-x

Immunogenetics of IgG4-Related AIP

Masao Ota, Takeji Umemura and Shigeyuki Kawa

Abstract Autoimmune pancreatitis (AIP) is a unique form of chronic pancreatitis characterized by high serum IgG4 concentration and a variety of complicating extra-pancreatic lesions. AIP has the features of a complex disease that is caused by multifactorial genes. However, the genetic factors underlying AIP have not been elucidated conclusively. Association studies by the candidate-gene approach and genome-wide association studies (GWAS) have revealed several susceptibility genes for AIP, including *HLA DRB1*04:05-DQB1*04:01*, *FCRL3*, *CTLA4*, and *KCNA3*, albeit in small-scale analyses. Thus, GWAS of large sample sizes and multinational collaborative meta-analyses are needed to identify the precise genetic variants that are associated with AIP onset. Systems genetics approaches that integrate DNA sequencing, expression quantitative trait locus (eQTL) mapping, proteomics, and metabolomics will also be useful in clarifying the pathogenesis of AIP.

Contents

M. Ota (✉)
Department of Legal Medicine, Shinshu University School of Medicine, Matsumoto, Japan
e-mail: otamasao@shinshu-u.ac.jp

T. Umemura
Department of Internal Medicine, Division of Gastroenterology and Hepatology, Shinshu University School of Medicine, Matsumoto, Japan

S. Kawa
Center for Health, Safety, and Environmental Management, Shinshu University, Matsumoto, Japan

Current Topics in Microbiology and Immunology (2017) 401: 35–44
DOI 10.1007/82_2016_37

Published Online: 10 November 2016

1 Introduction

Autoimmune pancreatitis (AIP) is a newly recognized pancreatic disorder characterized by lymphoplasmacytic inflammation, tissue infiltration IgG4-positive cells, elevated serum IgG4 concentration, a favorable response to corticosteroid treatment, and a variety of complicating extra-pancreatic lesions (Hamano et al. 2001, 2002; Yamamoto et al. 2005; Kamisawa et al. 2003; Masaki et al. 2009). AIP comprises two subtypes, type 1 and type 2, based on the clinical and pathological features (Shimosegawa et al. 2011; Sah et al. 2010). Type 1 AIP is typified by a male preponderance, elevated serum IgG4, and occurrence predominantly in Japan. This subtype is also recognized as a pancreatic manifestation of IgG4-related disease (IgG4-RD) (Kamisawa et al. 2010). The etiology and pathogenesis of type 1 AIP (hereafter referred to as AIP) remain largely unclear.

AIP phenotype is influenced by multiple immune-mediated mechanisms in addition to the environmental and genetic factors. Thus, this disorder may have the features of a complex disease that is caused by multifactorial genes. Although identifying these genes is complex, two approaches using case-control studies have been employed to elucidate the genetic factors that influence disease susceptibility (Amos et al. 2011): the candidate-gene approach by association studies and genome-wide association testing of large numbers of single nucleotide polymorphisms (SNPs). In the candidate-gene approach, an association study is carried out using polymorphic markers (SNPs and microsatellites) that reside around or within biologically functional genes presumably involved in disease development. When the fundamental pathophysiology of a disease is unknown, however, genome-wide studies are suitable to hunt down causative genes. Genome-wide association studies (GWAS) are a powerful and widely used technique for exploring the relationships among common sequence variations and disease susceptibility or resistance throughout the entire genome. Here, we summarize the recent advances of studies on the genetic predisposition to AIP, focusing particularly on data obtained from case-control studies in the Japanese population.

2 Association Studies Using Polymorphic Markers in Candidate Genes

2.1 Human Leukocyte Antigen (HLA) Complex

The HLA complex contains the most polymorphic genes in the human genome (Mungall et al. 2003). Genetic variations in HLA genes have been associated with susceptibility to autoimmune and infectious diseases (Shiina et al. 2009; Fernando et al. 2008) and play a major role in transplantation medicine and immunology. Furthermore, HLA class II genes have been genetically characterized as primary predisposition factors of AIP in Japan (Kawa et al. 2002; Ota et al. 2007). Recent association findings with HLA alleles after increasing the number of patients are shown in Table 1, where *HLA-DPB1* alleles are seen to have a negative association. HLA alleles with AIP were unsuccessful in a Korean population; however, a significant correlation was found between the absence of aspartic acid at codon 57 of DQβ1 and disease relapse (Park et al. 2008) that was not in the Japanese (Hirano et al. 2009). Elsewhere, Freitag et al. supported that the *HLA-DB1*04:05* allele was an important risk factor for AIP in functional studies using a transgenic mouse model (Freitag et al. 2010).

*2.2 Fc Receptor-Like 3 (*FCRL3*) Gene*

FCRL3 genes have high structural homology with classical Fcγ receptor genes. The FCRL3 protein is an orphan receptor preferentially expressed by B-lineage cells. A functional promoter −169 C/T polymorphism in the *FCRL3* gene has been linked to various autoimmune diseases, including rheumatoid arthritis, autoimmune thyroid disease, and systemic lupus erythematosus, in the Japanese population (Ikari et al. 2006). In our association analysis of AIP, four SNP markers (*FCRL3*

Table 1 Significant HLA alleles associated with AIP

HLA allele		AIP (n = 220) n (%)	Control (n = 386) n (%)	OR (95 % CI)	P	Pc
HLA-A*	02:06	7 (0.032)	41 (0.106)	0.28 (0.80–0.16)	0.0011	0.017
	24:02	72 (0.327)	86 (0.223)	1.70 (1.17–2.45)	0.0048	
HLA-DRB1*	04:05	62 (0.282)	52 (0.135)	2.52 (1.68–3.79)	0.0000084	0.00022
	13:02	29 (0.132)	29 (0.074)	1.87 (1.09–3.20)	0.0230	
HLA-DQB1*	04:01	61 (0.277)	49 (0.127)	2.64 (1.74–3.98)	0.0000039	0.000059

Table 2 Case-control analysis of *FCRL3* gene polymorphisms and AIP

FCRL3 SNP	Position	Allele	Minor Allele frequency *n* (%)		*P*	OR (95 % CI)
			AIP	Control		
fclr3_3, rs7528684	−169	T > C	(n = 124)	(n = 1298)	0.26	1.24 (0.85–1.81)
		CC/TC +TT	49 (39.5)	448 (34.5)	0.024	2.16 (1.09–4.26)
fclr3_4, rs11264799	−110	G > A	(n = 124)	(n = 1306)	0.0078	1.75 (1.15–2.65)
		AA/AG +GG	35 (28.2)	240 (18.4)	0.000013	5.90 (2.45–15.32)
fcrl3_5, rs945635	+358	G > C	(n = 124)	(n = 1260)	0.25	1.25 (0.85–1.82)
		GG/GC +CC	49 (39.5)	433 (34.4)	0.039	2.02 (1.02–3.98)
fclr3_6, rs3761959	+1381	G > A	(n = 124)	(n = 1260)	0.25	1.25 (0.85–1.82)
		GG/GA +AA	49 (39.5)	433 (34.4)	0.039	2.02 (1.02–3.98)

−169*C/T [*fclr3_3*, rs7528684], *FCR3* −110*A/G *[fclr3_4*, rs11264799], *FCRL3* +358*C/G [*fcrl3_5*, rs945635], and *FCRL3* +1381*A/G [*fclr3_6*, rs3761959]) provided the most significant P values without correction in recessive-trait genotype comparisons of *fcrl3_4* (*P* = 0.000013, OR = 5.90) (Table 2).

A positive correlation between the susceptibility allele A of *fcrl3_4* and serum titers of IgG4 antibodies has been found as well (Umemura et al. 2006). *FCRL3* gene polymorphisms modulate the gene expression through NF-κB binding. FCRL3 expression on B cells has been observed in significant amounts in individuals with the disease-susceptible genotype (Kochi et al. 2005). The augmented expression of *FCRL3* seems to be associated with susceptibility to AIP disorders.

*2.3 Cytotoxic T-Lymphocyte Antigen-4 (*CTLA-4; CD152*) Gene*

One of the characteristic pathological features of AIP is lymphoplasmacytic infiltration of immune cells, including CD4- and CD8-positive T cells and IgG4-producing plasma cells, into the pancreatic parenchyma and other involved organs. Thus, factors regulating T-cell function are likely involved in the development of AIP. CTLA-4 (CD152) is an inhibitory receptor expressed on activated memory T cells (CD4+ CD25+ regulatory T cells) and acts largely as a negative regulator of T-cell responses (Gough et al. 2005). A significant association of *CTLA-4* gene polymorphisms (+49A/G SNP, +6230G/A) with various autoimmune diseases has been described (Ueda et al. 2003). In Japanese patients, the +6230 SNP in the 3′ untranslated region of *CTLA-4* played a critical role in both susceptibility to and protection from AIP (Umemura et al. 2008). Moreover, a significant increase in the

Table 3 Case-control analysis of *CTLA-4* gene polymorphisms and AIP

CTLA-4	Allele	Major allele frequency n (%)		P	OR
		AIP (n = 59)	Control (n = 102)		
+6230	G > A GG/AA+AG	92 (78.0)	133 (65.2)	0.016 0.0065	1.89 (1.12–3.18) 2.48 (1.28–4.81)
+49	G > A	77 (65.8)	113 (55.4)	0.08	1.51 (0.95–2.41)
−318	C > T	101 (85.6)	184 (90.2)	0.21	0.64 (0.32–1.28)
−1722	T > C	72 (61.0)	72 (61.0)	0.51	0.85 (0.53–1.36)

+6230 G/G genotype (P = 0.007, OR = 2.48) was found in Japanese AIP patients (Table 3). In Taiwanese patients with AIP, the *CTLA-4* +49 A allele in exon 1 exhibited significantly higher frequencies than in healthy individuals (Chang et al. 2007). The incidence of +6230A in various haplotypes (−1722, −658, −318, +49, and +6230) has been associated with AIP resistance (P = 0.011, OR = 0.49) (Umemura et al. 2008).

2.4 *Toll-Like Receptor 4 (TLR4) and Protein Tyrosine Phosphatase N22 (PTPN22) Genes*

Many autoimmune diseases cause similar pathological features and have a tendency to share common susceptibility genes in disease development (Gregersen and Behrens 2006). Among them, TLR4 has been the most thoroughly investigated among autoimmune diseases (Akira et al. 2006). TLR4 is a transmembrane protein expressed by the cells of the innate immune system that recognizes pathogen-associated molecular patterns and is essential in immune and inflammatory responses to pathogenic invaders. In our association study, however, *TLR4* polymorphisms did not factor significantly in the etiology of AIP (Umemura et al. 2009).

The *PTPN22* gene encodes a lymphoid-specific protein tyrosine phosphatase (Lyp) that is important in the control of T-cell activation and in T-cell development. A missense SNP known as rs2476601 in *PTPN22* has been consistently associated with a variety of autoimmune diseases (Burn et al. 2011). Although *PTPN22* seems to be a general susceptibility locus for autoimmunity, it is not involved in predisposition to AIP (Table 4).

AIP appears to have a complex genetic background wherein multiple genes contribute to disease risk with modest independent effect. Candidate-gene approaches using association studies with polymorphic markers have succeeded in identifying several causal genes for the disorder. However, candidate-gene case-control studies often suffer from insufficient statistical power owing to

Table 4 Allelic association tests of 7 genotyped SNPs in *PTPN22*

SNP	Position on Chr. 13	Allele	Minor allele frequency (%)		*P* value	OR (95 % CI)
			Controls (n = 322)	AIP (n = 127)		
rs1217412	113814589	G > A	42.4	41.7	0.86	0.97 (0.73–1.31)
rs1217388	113821854	G > A	42.4	41.7	0.86	0.97 (0.73–1.31)
rs1217407	113851126	A > G	42.4	41.7	0.86	0.97 (0.73–1.31)
rs3765598	113851841	C > T	21.6	22.1	0.88	1.03 (0.72–1.46)
rs2488458	113863829	T > C	42.4	41.7	0.86	0.97 (0.73–1.31)
rs3789612	113871486	C > T	8.5	9.5	0.67	1.12 (0.68–1.85)
rs2488457	113872746	G > C	42.2	42.1	0.97	1.00 (0.74–1.34)

inadequate sample size. On that point, GWAS requiring hundreds of thousands of genetic markers and thousands of individuals provide much greater power to reveal disease-causative genes.

3 Association Studies Using Genome-Wide Polymorphic Markers

3.1 Microsatellite Markers

In a genomic microsatellite analysis using 400 microsatellite markers with an average spacing of 10.8 cM, the most significant association was found for the D1S2726 marker at the potassium voltage-gated channel, shaker-related subfamily, member 3 (*KCNA3*) gene (Table 5). Further association studies using SNPs surrounding the *KCNA3* gene confirmed a possible association of *KCNA3* with AIP and influence on AIP risk (Ota et al. 2011). KCNA3 is involved in the immune modulation of auto-reactive effector and memory T cell-mediated autoimmune diseases (Beeton et al. 2006).

3.2 Small-Scale GWAS for Detecting Genetic Factors Causing the Development of Lachrymal/Salivary Gland Lesions in AIP

Patients with AIP often suffer from a variety of complicating extra-pancreatic lesions. Dacryoadenitis/sialadenitis is one of such manifestations that is now considered to be a principal feature of IgG4-RD (Stone et al. 2012). Lachrymal/salivary gland lesions tend to appear in a highly active AIP disease state, and several genes

Table 5 Association of KCNA3 SNPs and D1S2726 microsatellite marker with AIP

Chromosome	Locus	Allele	AIP % ($n = 64$)	Control % ($n = 104$)	OR	95 % CI	*P*
1	D1S2726	280	42.2	8.7	7.7	3.3–17.9	0.00000074
	D1S0655i	266	73.4	45.2	3.4	1.7–6.6	0.00034

Chromosome	KCNA3 SNP	Allele 1/2	Major allele frequency		OR	95 % CI	*P*
			AIP % ($n = 128$)	Cont % (208)			
1	rs3762379	C/T	99.2	85.6	1.99	0.94–4.22	0.0692
	rs2821557	C/T	64.8	56.7	1.14	0.89–2.22	0.1407
	rs2840381	G/A	59.4	43.8	1.88	1.20–2.94	0.0054
	rs1058184	A/C	56.3	40.9	1.86	1.19–2.90	0.0061
	rs2640480	C/A	56.3	40.9	1.86	1.19–2.90	0.0061
	rs1319782	C/T	56.3	40.9	1.86	1.19–2.90	0.0061
	rs2821548	G/A	60.9	55.3	1.26	0.81–1.97	0.3091
	rs3887820	C/A	58.6	45.7	1.68	1.08–2.63	0.0214

are speculated to be associated with the onset of this complication. To identify the candidate susceptibility genes related to lachrymal/salivary gland lesions, we first carried out GWAS using the GeneChip Human Mapping 500 k Array Set (Affymetrix, CA) as a screening step. Next, fine-tuned mapping of specific SNPs was performed for candidate genes that showed a strong statistical significance ($P < 0.0001$). A total of four genes (*KLF7*, *FTMD4B*, *NOX3*, and *MPPED2*) were determined as candidate genes involved in the development of lachrymal/salivary gland lesions in AIP (Oguchi et al. 2015).

Terao et al. performed GWAS by genotyping 2,310,564 SNPs in 850 patients with AIP, IgG-related sialadenitis, or IgG-related kidney diseases and in 2082 healthy individuals. They proposed that the *FCGR2B* gene and *HLA-DRB1* amino acid position 11 have an important role in the development and progression of IgG4-RD [abstract in EULAR 2016].

4 Conclusions and Future Perspectives

The AIP phenotype appears to be influenced by diverse genetic, environmental, and cultural factors. To date, association studies by the candidate-gene approach and small-scale GWAS have several susceptibility genes, including HLA *DRB1*04:05-DQB1*04:01*, *FCRL3*, *CTLA4*, and *KCNA3*. However, disease susceptibility remains poorly understood for AIP. Although GWAS are a powerful tool to uncover numerous common variants that contribute to disease predisposition in complex diseases, no GWAS of a large sample size and well-defined cohort using precise clinical diagnostic criteria have been done on AIP. If the study is to be performed on a small scale, a replication test using a larger sample size and meta-analysis by multinational collaboration may also elucidate the heterogeneity of genetic risk factors. Given the earlier progress in the identification of susceptibility genes by GWAS, the next steps will be toward understanding how these risk genes are regulated using fine-mapping studies and next generation sequencing methods for candidate genes, whole exomes, and even genomes if available.

Lastly, it is possible that differences in gene expression levels may be involved in phenotypic variation and susceptibility to AIP as well. Expression quantitative trait locus mapping is useful in determining the effects of genetic variants on gene expression levels (Fairfax and Knight 2014). Further studies employing systems genetics approaches (Civelek and Lusis 2014), including DNA sequencing, proteomics, and metabolomics, are expected to shed light on the pathogenesis of AIP.

References

Akira S, Uematsu S, Takeuchi O (2006) Pathogen recognition and innate immunity. Cell 124 (4):783–801. doi:10.1016/j.cell.2006.02.015

Amos W, Driscoll E, Hoffman JI (2011) Candidate genes versus genome-wide associations: which are better for detecting genetic susceptibility to infectious disease? Proc Biol Sci 278 (1709):1183–1188. doi:10.1098/rspb

Beeton C, Wulff H, Standifer NE, Azam P, Mullen KM et al (2006) Kv1.3 channels are a therapeutic target for T cell-mediated autoimmune diseases. Proc Natl Acad Sci USA 103 (46):17414–17419. doi:10.1073/pnas.0605136103

Burn GL, Svensson L, Sanchez-Blanco C, Saini M, Cope AP (2011) Why is PTPN22 a good candidate susceptibility gene for autoimmune disease? FEBS Lett 585(23):3689–3698. doi:10.1016/j.febslet

Chang MC, Chang YT, Tien YW, Liang PC, Jan IS, Wei SC, Wong JM (2007) T-cell regulatory gene CTLA-4 polymorphism/haplotype association with autoimmune pancreatitis. Clin Chem 53(9):1700–1705. doi:10.1373/clinchem.2007.085951

Civelek M, Lusis AJ (2014) Systems genetics approaches to understand complex traits. Nat Rev Genet 15(1):34–48. doi:10.1038/nrg3575

Fairfax BP, Knight JC (2014) Genetics of gene expression in immunity to infection. Curr Opin Immunol 30:63–71. doi:10.1016/j.coi.2014.07.001

Fernando MM, Stevens CR, Walsh EC, De Jager PL, Goyette P, Plenge RM, Vyse TJ, Rioux JD (2008) Defining the role of the MHC in autoimmunity: a review and pooled analysis. PLoS Genet: e1000024. doi:10.1371/journal.pgen.1000024

Freitag TL, Cham C, Sung HH, Beilhack GF, Durinovic-Belló I, Patel SD, Bronson RT, Schuppan D, Sønderstrup G (2010) Human risk allele HLA-DRB1*0405 predisposes class II transgenic Ab0 NOD mice to autoimmune pancreatitis. Gastroenterology 139(1):281–291. doi:10.1053/j.gastro.2010.03.038

Gough SC, Walker LS, Sansom DM (2005) CTLA4gene polymorphism and autoimmunity. Immunol Rev 204:102–115. doi:10.1111/j.0105-2896.2005.00249.x

Gregersen PK, Behrens TW (2006) Genetics of autoimmune diseases–disorders of immune homeostasis. Nat Rev Genet 7(12):917–928. doi:10.1038/nrg1944

Hamano H, Kawa S, Horiuchi A, Unno H, Furuya N, Akamatsu T, Fukushima M, Nikaido T, Nakayama K, Usuda N, Kiyosawa K (2001) High serum IgG4 concentrations in patients with sclerosing pancreatitis. N Engl J Med 344(10):732–738. doi:10.1056/NEJM200103083441005

Hamano H, Kawa S, Ochi Y, Unno H, Shiba N, Wajiki M, Nakazawa K, Shimojo H, Kiyosawa K (2002) Hydronephrosis associated with retroperitoneal fibrosis and sclerosing pancreatitis. Lancet 20(359):1403–1404. doi:10.1016/S0140-6736(02)08359-9
Hirano K, Asaoka Y, Tada M, Isayama H, Sasahira N, Tsujino T, Kawabe T, Omata M (2009) No significant relation between relapse of autoimmune pancreatitis and substitution of aspartic acid at position 57 of DQbeta1. J Gastroenterol 44(7):799–800. doi:10.1007/s00535-009-0080-4
Ikari K, Momohara S, Nakamura T, Hara M, Yamanaka H, Tomatsu T, Kamatani N (2006) Supportive evidence for a genetic association of the FCRL3 promoter polymorphism with rheumatoid arthritis. Ann Rheum Dis 65(5):671–673. doi:10.1136/ard.2005.043489
Kamisawa T, Funata N, Hayashi Y, Tsuruta K, Okamoto A, Amemiya K, Egawa N, Nakajima H (2003) Close relationship between autoimmune pancreatitis and multifocal fibrosclerosis. Gut 52(5):683–687. doi:10.1136/gut.52.5.683
Kamisawa T, Notohara K, Shimosegawa T (2010) Two clinicopathologic subtypes of autoimmune pancreatitis: LPSP and IDCP. Gastroenterology 139(1):22–25. doi:10.1053/j.gastro.2010.05.019
Kawa S, Ota M, Yoshizawa K, Horiuchi A, Hamano H, Ochi Y, Nakayama K, Tokutake Y, Katsuyama Y, Saito S, Hasebe O, Kiyosawa K (2002) HLA DRB10405-DQB10401 haplotype is associated with autoimmune pancreatitis in the Japanese population. Gastroenterology 122 (5):1264–1269. doi:10.1053/gast.2002.33022
Kochi Y, Yamada R, Suzuki A, Harley JB, Shirasawa S, Sawada T, Bae SC, Tokuhiro S, Chang X, Sekine A, Takahashi A, Tsunoda T, Ohnishi Y, Kaufman KM, Kang CP, Kang C, Otsubo S, Yumura W, Mimori A, Koike T, Nakamura Y, Sasazuki T, Yamamoto K (2005) A functional variant in FCRL3, encoding Fc receptor-like 3, is associated with rheumatoid arthritis and several autoimmunities. Nat Genet 37(5):478–485. doi:10.1038/ng1540
Masaki Y, Dong L, Kurose N, Kitagawa K, Morikawa Y, Yamamoto M, Takahashi H, Shinomura Y, Imai K, Saeki T, Azumi A, Nakada S, Sugiyama E, Matsui S, Origuchi T, Nishiyama S, Nishimori I, Nojima T, Yamada K, Kawano M, Zen Y, Kaneko M, Miyazaki K, Tsubota K, Eguchi K, Tomoda K, Sawaki T, Kawanami T, Tanaka M, Fukushima T, Sugai S, Umehara H (2009) Proposal for a new clinical entity, IgG4-positive multiorgan lymphoproliferative syndrome: analysis of 64 cases of IgG4-related disorders. Ann Rheum Dis 68 (8):1310–1315. doi:10.1136/ard.2008.089169
Mungall AJ, Palmer SA, Sims SK, Edwards CA, Ashurst JL et al (2003) The DNA sequence and analysis of human chromosome 6. Nature 425(6960):805–811. doi:10.1038/nature02055
Oguchi T, Ota M, Ito T, Hamano H, Arakura N, Katsuyama Y, Meguro A, Kawa S. (2015) Investigation of susceptibility genes triggering lachrymal/salivary gland lesion complications in Japanese patients with type 1 autoimmune pancreatitis. PLoS One: e0127078. doi:10.1371/journal.pone.0127078 (eCollection 2016;11(1):e0146738. doi:10.1371/journal.pone.0146738)
Ota M, Katsuyama Y, Hamano H, Umemura T, Kimura A, Yoshizawa K, Kiyosawa K, Fukushima H, Bahram S, Inoko H, Kawa S (2007) Two critical genes (HLA-DRB1 and ABCF1) in the HLA region are associated with the susceptibility to autoimmune pancreatitis. Immunogenetics 59(1):45–52. doi:10.1007/s00251-006-0178-2
Ota M, Ito T, Umemura T, Katsuyama Y, Yoshizawa K, Hamano H, Kawa S (2011) Polymorphism in the KCNA3 gene is associated with susceptibility to autoimmune pancreatitis in the Japanese population. Dis Markers 31(4):223–229. doi:10.3233/DMA-2011-0820
Park DH, Kim MH, Oh HB, Kwon OJ, Choi YJ, Lee SS, Lee TY, Seo DW, Lee SK (2008) Substitution of aspartic acid at position 57 of the DQbeta1 affects relapse of autoimmune pancreatitis. Gastroenterology 134(2):440–446. doi:10.1053/j.gastro.2007.11.023
Sah RP, Chari ST, Pannala R, Sugumar A, Clain JE, Levy MJ, Pearson RK, Smyrk TC, Petersen BT, Topazian MD, Takahashi N, Farnell MB, Vege SS (2010) Differences in clinical profile and relapse rate of type 1 versus type 2 autoimmune pancreatitis. Gastroenterology 139 (1):140–148. doi:10.1053/j.gastro.2010.03.054
Shiina T, Hosomichi K, Inoko H, Kulski JK (2009) The HLA genomic loci map: expression, interaction, diversity and disease. J Hum Genet 54(1):15–39. doi:10.1038/jhg.2008.5

Shimosegawa T, Chari ST, Frulloni L, Kamisawa T, Kawa S, Mino-Kenudson M, Kim MH, Klöppel G, Lerch MM, Löhr M, Notohara K, Okazaki K, Schneider A, Zhang L; International Association of Pancreatology (2011) International consensus diagnostic criteria for autoimmune pancreatitis: guidelines of the International Association of Pancreatology. Pancreas 40 (3):352–358. doi:10.1097/MPA.0b013e3182142fd2

Stone JH, Khosroshahi A, Deshpande V, Chan JK, Heathcote JG et al (2012) Recommendations for the nomenclature of IgG4-related disease and its individual organ system manifestations. Arthritis Rheum 64:3061–3067. doi:10.1002/art.34593

Ueda H, Howson JM, Esposito L, Heward J, Snook H, et al (2003) Association of the T-cell regulatory gene CTLA4 with susceptibility to autoimmune disease. Nature 423(6939):506–511. doi:10.1038/nature01621

Umemura T, Ota M, Hamano H, Katsuyama Y, Kiyosawa K, Kawa S (2006) Genetic association of Fc receptor-like 3 polymorphisms with autoimmune pancreatitis in Japanese patients. Gut 55 (9):1367–1368. doi:10.1136/gut.2006.095059

Umemura T, Ota M, Hamano H, Katsuyama Y, Muraki T, Arakura N, Kawa S, Kiyosawa K (2008) Association of autoimmune pancreatitis with cytotoxic T-lymphocyte antigen 4 gene polymorphisms in Japanese patients. Am J Gastroenterol 103(3):588–594. doi:10.1111/j.1572-0241

Umemura T, Katsuyama Y, Hamano H, Kitahara K, Takayama M, Arakura N, Kawa S, Tanaka E, Ota M (2009) Association analysis of Toll-like receptor 4 polymorphisms with autoimmune pancreatitis. Hum Immunol 70(9):742–746. doi:10.1016/j.humimm.2009.05.009

Yamamoto M, Harada S, Ohara M, Suzuki C, Naishiro Y, Yamamoto H, Takahashi H, Imai K (2005) Clinical and pathological differences between Mikulicz's disease and Sjögren's syndrome. Rheumatology 44(2):227–234. doi:10.1093/rheumatology/keh447

The Histopathology of IgG4-Related Disease

Mehmet Ozgur Avincsal and Yoh Zen

Abstract IgG4-related disease is a multi-organ immune-mediated chronic fibroinflammatory condition characterized by elevated serum IgG4 concentrations, tumefaction, and tissue infiltration by IgG4-positive plasma cells. The exact etiology of IgG4-related disease remains unclear with no known role of the IgG4 molecule itself being identified. Although the pancreas and salivary glands are the main organs affected, the involvement of other organs has also been reported. This multi-organ disease mimics a large number of malignant, infectious, and inflammatory disorders; therefore, a prompt differential diagnosis is important for selecting the right therapeutic strategy. Early steroid therapy assists in preventing tissue fibrosis, parenchymal extinction, and severe functional impairments in the affected organs. The definitive and prompt diagnosis of IgG4-related disease requires both histopathological confirmation and clinicopathological correlations. A histopathological examination is mandatory to exclude neoplastic or inflammatory conditions that mimic IgG4-related disease. The histological changes that occur are basically similar in any organ manifestation, with several site-specific findings being recognized. This chapter summarizes general rules for the pathological examination of IgG4-related disease, as well as the histopathological features and differential diagnoses of major organ manifestations.

M.O. Avincsal · Y. Zen (✉)
Department of Diagnostic Pathology, Kobe University Graduate School of Medicine, 7-5-2 Kusunoki-Cho, Kobe 650-0017, Japan
e-mail: yohzen@med.kobe-u.ac.jp

M.O. Avincsal
Department of Otolaryngology, Kobe University Graduate School of Medicine, Kobe, Japan

Current Topics in Microbiology and Immunology (2017) 401: 45–60
DOI 10.1007/82_2016_38

Published Online: 14 November 2016

Contents

1 Diagnosis of IgG4-Related Disease

IgG4-related disease (IgG4-RD) is a multi-organ immune-mediated chronic fibroinflammatory condition in which various organ manifestations are linked by a similar histological appearance (Stone et al. 2012). It is characterized by mass-forming sclerosing lesions, elevated serum IgG4 concentrations, and extensive tissue infiltration by IgG4 plasma cells (Hamano et al. 2001, 2002). Since the first report of patients with elevated serum IgG4 levels and autoimmune pancreatitis in 2001 (Hamano et al. 2001), neither the exact etiology of IgG4-RD nor the roles of the IgG4 molecule itself in the pathogenetic process have been elucidated. Although this multi-organ condition has now been described in almost every organ system, the majority of patients have at least one of pancreatitis, sialadenitis, dacryoadenitis, periaortitis, and interstitial nephritis (Inoue et al. 2015). Regardless of the organ involved, fibrosis and impaired function are the common outcomes of long-standing IgG4-related inflammation when left untreated. Furthermore, this multi-organ condition may mimic a large number of malignant, infectious, and inflammatory disorders. A prompt diagnosis is important because it typically responds to immunosuppressive therapy, thereby avoiding unnecessary invasive procedures.

The diagnosis of IgG4-RD involves a combination of clinical, radiological, serological, and histopathological features. A tissue examination is not essential for IgG4-related autoimmune pancreatitis because its imaging features are highly specific for this condition (Shimosegawa et al. 2011). In contrast, a histological diagnosis is crucial for manifestations in other organs. A caveat is that a tissue diagnosis is not always conclusive; therefore, careful clinicopathological correlations are required before establishing a definite diagnosis (Deshpande et al. 2012).

2 General Pathological Features of IgG4-RD

2.1 Morphological Features

According to the consensus statement on the pathology of IgG4-RD published in 2012 (Deshpande et al. 2012), a tissue diagnosis of IgG4-RD needs to be based on both morphological and immunohistochemical findings regardless of the organs involved. Three characteristic morphological findings of IgG-RD are diffuse lymphoplasmacytic infiltration, storiform fibrosis, and obliterative phlebitis.

Dense lymphoplasmacytic infiltrate: In the first stage, affected tissues are diffusely and densely infiltrated by lymphoplasmacytic cells (Fig. 1a). The lymphocytic infiltrate is composed predominantly of T cells, with scattered aggregates of B cells. Lymphoid follicle formation may occur, and it is particularly common in sialadenitis and dacryoadenitis (Zen and Nakanuma 2010). Plasma cells are also abundant and occasionally arranged in sheets. Infiltrating plasma cells are polyclonal in nature. B cells with variable differentiation such as immunoblasts may also be identifiable.

Storiform fibrosis: In the second stage, fibrosis ensues from fibroblasts found in the lymphoplasmacytic infiltrate and is characteristically arranged in a storiform

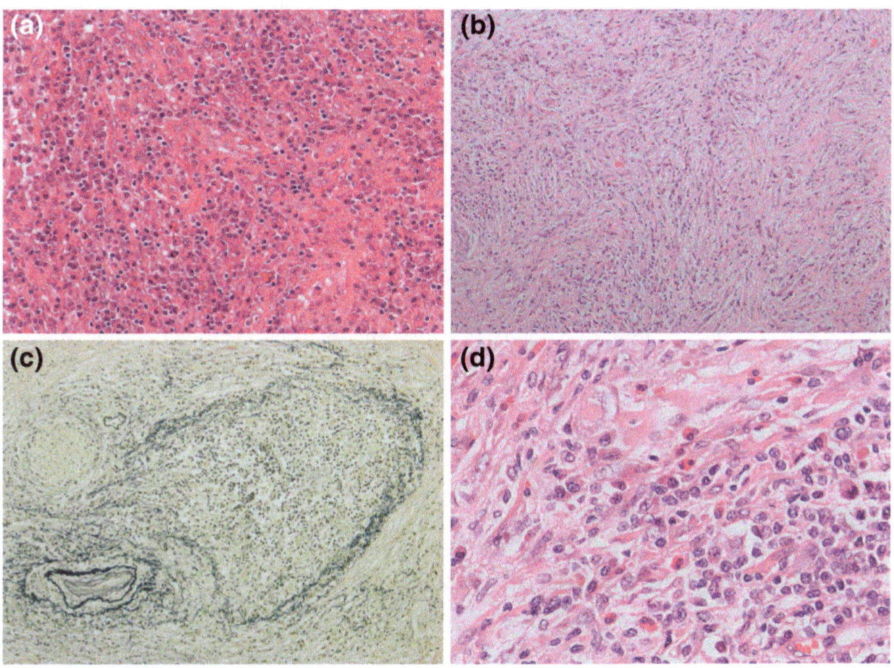

Fig. 1 Characteristic histological features of IgG4-RD. **a** A massive lymphoplasmacytic infiltration is observed against the background of little fibrosis. **b** Collagen fibers are arranged in a storiform pattern. **c** Elastica van Gieson staining reveals an obliterated vein (obliterative phlebitis). **d** Occasional eosinophils are present

pattern (Fig. 1b). Some degree of fibrosis may be present even in the earliest stage of the disease. Storiform fibrosis consists of collagen fibers arranged in an irregularly whorled pattern, somewhat resembling the spokes of a cartwheel or the net of a straw mat. A caveat is that the standard for this form of fibrosis appears to vary among pathologists, with no universally accepted definition currently being available. The storiform pattern of fibrosis may not be detected in limited samples such as needle biopsies. Furthermore, the severity of fibrosis depends on the individual organs involved. For example, storiform fibrosis is characteristic of IgG4-related autoimmune pancreatitis or retroperitoneal fibrosis, but is less commonly found in patients with IgG4-related dacryoadenitis or lymphadenopathy (Zen and Nakanuma 2010).

Obliterative phlebitis: Venous channels are partially or completely obliterated by the dense lymphoplasmacytic infiltrate and fibrosis (Fig. 1c). Lymphocytes and plasma cells are detected within the wall of the venous channel and within the lumina of small- and medium-sized veins. The presence of obliterative phlebitis needs to be established thoroughly because of its diagnostic value, ideally through the use of elastin stains targeting the elastic lamina of the vessel. In contrast to systemic vasculitides such as granulomatosis with polyangiitis, microscopic polyangiitis, polyarteritis nodosa, and leukocytoclastic vasculitis, necrosis of the vascular wall and fibrin deposition are not observed in IgG4-RD.

Other findings: Eosinophils are commonly present, and extreme examples may resemble eosinophilic organopathy (e.g., eosinophilic cholangitis) (Fig. 1d). Macrophages are also typically detectable within the fibroinflammatory infiltrate and are highlighted by immunostaining for CD163, a marker for M2-type macrophages (Zen et al. 2015). Arteritis is occasionally observed in cases of IgG4-related lung disease (Zen et al. 2005, 2009a). Arteritis associated with IgG4-related disease is characterized by a non-necrotizing lymphoplasmacytic infiltrate with or without the obliteration of the lumen, similar to obliterative phlebitis.

Findings against the diagnosis of IgG4-RD: Several histological changes are known to seldom occur in this condition. It is important to confirm that these findings are not present before reaching a diagnosis of IgG4-RD because these "negative" findings suggest an alternative diagnosis. Despite the massive inflammatory infiltrate, neutrophils are rare in IgG4-RD. Necrosis is not expected at any stage of disease progression. Although macrophages are present, a xanthogranulomatous change, epithelioid granulomata, and giant cells are unusual for this condition (Zen and Nakanuma 2010; Deshpande et al. 2012).

2.2 Immunohistochemical Features

High numbers of IgG4-positive plasma cells at tissue sites are a disease hallmark, even when serum IgG4 concentrations are normal (Fig. 2). This finding is helpful for differentiating IgG4-RD from other plasma cell-rich disorders, such as primary sclerosing cholangitis and multicentric Castleman's disease (Kamisawa et al. 2014). Immunohistochemistry with IgG4 staining is a highly reproducible method to

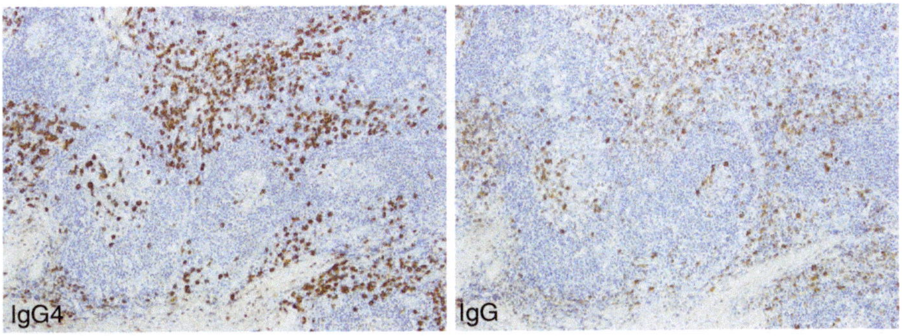

Fig. 2 Immunohistochemical findings of IgG4-RD. Many IgG4-positive plasma cells are observed (*left*). Compared to IgG-positive plasma cells (*right*), the ratio of IgG4/IgG-positive plasma cells appears to be greater than 40 %

Table 1 Cutoff points for IgG4-positive plasma cell counts in various organs

Meningus	>10
Lacrimal gland	>100
Salivary gland	>100
Lymph node	>100
Lung (surgical specimen)	>50
Lung (biopsy)	>20
Pleura	>50
Pancreas (surgical specimen)	>50
Pancreas (biopsy)	>10
Bile duct (surgical specimen)	>50
Bile duct (biopsy)	>10
Liver (surgical specimen)	>50
Liver (biopsy)	>10
Kidney (surgical specimen)	>30
Kidney (biopsy)	>10
Aorta	>50
Retroperitoneum	>30
Skin	>200

identify IgG4-positive plasma cells and needs to be performed in all suspected cases of this condition. Since IgG4-positive plasma cells may be found in other inflammatory, neoplastic, and infectious conditions, various cutoff points, ranging from more than 10 to more than 100 IgG4-positive plasma cells per high-power field, have been proposed for individual organ manifestations in order to increase the diagnostic accuracy of the immunohistochemical examination. (Table 1) (Deshpande et al. 2012). The ratio of IgG4-positive plasma cells to IgG-positive plasma cells further assists in confirming the diagnosis of IgG4-RD (Fig. 2). A ratio higher than 40 % is very suggestive of the diagnosis.

3 Proposed Diagnostic Terminology for IgG4-RD

Appropriate histopathological findings are essential, but not sufficient to establish a diagnosis. Clinicopathological correlations need to be performed before a definite diagnosis is reached. The 2012 Boston criteria provide guidance as to the level of confidence of a diagnosis of IgG4-RD based on histopathological examinations of tissue samples. The consensus statement proposes the following pathological classifications (Deshpande et al. 2012):

(1) Highly suggestive of disease
(2) Probable histological features of disease
(3) Insufficient evidence of IgG4-RD.

Histology highly suggestive of IgG4-RD requires at least two histopathological features, which include a dense lymphoplasmacytic infiltrate, storiform fibrosis, and obliterative phlebitis. In addition, an increased number of IgG4-positive plasma cells greater than the cutoff point and an elevated IgG4/IgG cell ratio of more than 40 % need to be proven. If a pathology specimen meets only one morphological feature and immunohistochemical criteria, the case is said to have probable histological features of the disease. In this situation, additional evidence (e.g., serum IgG4 level greater than 135 mg/dL and other organ involvement) needs to be confirmed for a diagnosis. If the criteria from either category are unable to be met, the case has insufficient evidence of IgG4-RD.

The histological features of IgG4-RD are broadly similar across the various organs and organ systems, but some pathological differences exist. For example, storiform fibrosis and obliterative phlebitis are not common in some organs, while arterial involvement is unique in lung lesions (Zen and Nakanuma 2010). The histological changes in these organs may mimic other diseases that are prevalent at the particular anatomical sites. Histopathological features and pathological differential diagnoses of major organ manifestations are discussed below.

4 Pancreatobiliary Manifestations

Major manifestations in these organ systems are type 1 autoimmune pancreatitis, sclerosing cholangitis, and an inflammatory pseudotumor of the liver (Zen et al. 2016; Okazaki and Uchida 2015; Hart et al. 2015). IgG4-RD at these anatomical sites produces prototypic histopathological features with no site-specific changes.

A major clinical differential diagnosis of IgG4-related pancreatitis is ductal adenocarcinoma of the pancreas, while a histological differential diagnosis includes other forms of chronic pancreatitis. Chronic alcoholic pancreatitis is generally a more fibrotic process with less severe lymphoplasmacytic infiltration and more extensive acinar atrophy than IgG4-related pancreatitis. Ductal changes such as duct ectasia or ulceration are more common in alcoholic pancreatitis. Type 2 autoimmune pancreatitis and follicular pancreatitis are histological mimics of IgG4-RD (Zen et al. 2012b; Zamboni et al. 2004; Notohara et al. 2003). A diagnosis of type 2 autoimmune pancreatitis requires a tissue confirmation of granulocytic epithelial lesions and extensive neutrophilic lobular inflammation, both of which are unlikely to occur in IgG4-related pancreatitis (Zhang et al. 2011). Follicular pancreatitis is a rare form of idiopathic pancreatitis, which has been called pseudolymphoma or reactive lymphoid hyperplasia of the pancreas. It is characterized by the formation of a large number of lymphoid follicles around pancreatic ducts (Zen et al. 2012b). Follicular pancreatitis is a less fibrotic process than IgG4-related pancreatitis, with only a small number of IgG4-positive plasma cells.

IgG4-related sclerosing cholangitis presents with either diffuse cholangiopathy mimicking primary sclerosing cholangitis (PSC) or periductal mass lesions resembling hilar cholangiocarcinoma. Although the clinical picture of IgG4-related sclerosing cholangitis may mimic PSC, their histological changes differ significantly. PSC is characterized by epithelial injury (e.g., ulceration and ductopenia), the fibroobliteration of bile ducts, and xanthogranulomatous inflammation, all of which are uncommon in IgG4-related sclerosing cholangitis (Zen et al. 2004). IgG4-positive plasma cells may be present in bile ducts affected by PSC; however, their number and ratio to IgG-positive plasma cells are markedly smaller than those in IgG4-related sclerosing cholangitis. Thus, the presence of fibroobliterative changes including periductal concentric fibrosis and ductopenia in liver biopsies suggests PSC over IgG4-related cholangitis, while tissue infiltration by IgG4-positive plasma cells (>10 cells/hpf) favors IgG4-related cholangiopathy (Zen et al. 2012d; Umemura et al. 2007; Deshpande et al. 2009). It is important to note that hepatic inflammatory pseudotumors are not always IgG4-related. Inflammatory pseudotumors of the liver may be classified into lymphoplasmacytic and fibrohistiocytic types (Zen et al. 2007). The former is IgG4-related, whereas the latter is not. Non-IgG4-related fibrohistiocytic lesions are characterized by intraparenchymal mass lesions, xanthogranulomatous inflammation, and suppurative inflammation with neutrophilic aggregates. Some non-IgG4-related cases are supposedly caused by infection. Other uncommon differential diagnoses include follicular cholangitis and sclerosing cholangitis with granulocytic epithelial lesions, both of which are recently described conditions (Zen et al. 2012a, b).

5 Sialadenitis and Dacryoadenitis

Multi-gland involvement is common at this anatomical site (Kitagawa et al. 2005). Affected organs are diffusely enlarged with a massive inflammatory infiltrate and fibrosis. IgG4-related dacryoadenitis differs from other organ lesions in that fibrosis does not have a storiform pattern, whereas "patternless" fibrosis is frequently identified (Fig. 3). Obliterative phlebitis is also uncommon in IgG4-related

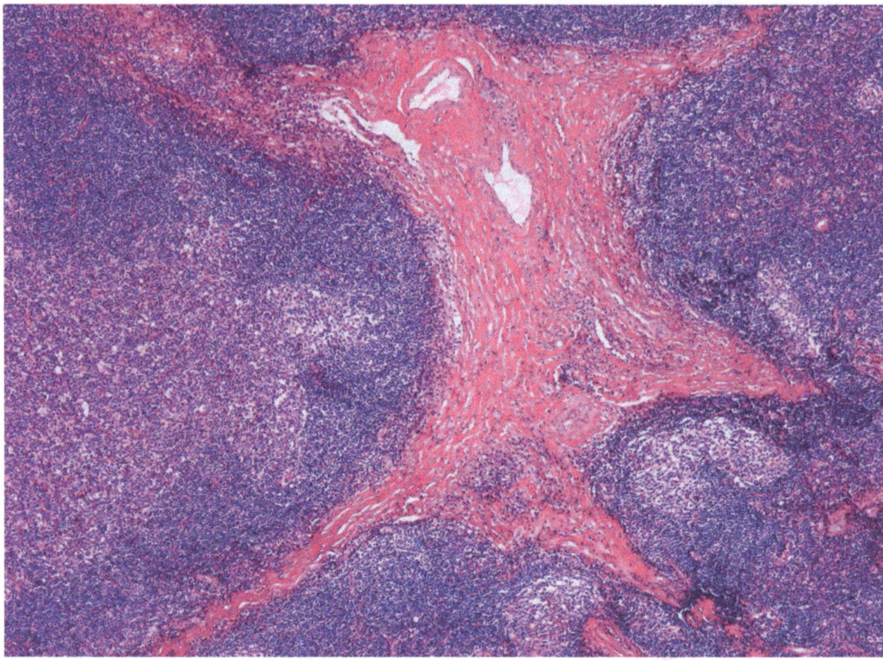

Fig. 3 IgG4-related dacryoadenitis. Densely collagenized fibrosis is observed. This pattern of fibrosis is less common in other organs

sialadenitis and dacryoadenitis. Many cases show only a dense lymphoplasmacytic infiltrate associated with large reactive germinal centers. Thus, the diagnosis of IgG4-RD at these anatomical sites relies on the presence of elevated numbers of IgG4-positive plasma cells and an IgG4 to IgG ratio of >40 %.

Major and minor salivary glands may both be affected by IgG4-RD. Sclerosis is more pronounced between acini, while inflammatory infiltration is more obvious inside the parenchyma. A differential diagnosis of IgG4-RD at this anatomical site is Sjögren syndrome (Yamamoto et al. 2005). This discrimination is relatively straightforward on clinical grounds (e.g., age and serological tests for SS-A or SS-B). Although IgG4-RD and Sjögren syndrome show marked lymphocytic infiltration, IgG4-RD is characterized by the formation of lymphoid follicles and less conspicuous duct injury. The absence of lymphoepithelial lesions in patients with IgG4-RD, in contrast to Sjögren syndrome, may explain the lower rate of dryness in the former, despite the marked swelling of lachrymal and salivary glands, and may also explain IgG4-RD xerostomia being improved by immunosuppression.

Another differential diagnosis is marginal zone B cell lymphoma of the MALT type (MALToma). It sometimes develops in the salivary gland with or without a previous history of Sjögren syndrome. Some cases of MALToma at this anatomical site consist of neoplastic cells with the IgG4 class switch (Sato et al. 2008).

Therefore, IgG4 immunostaining shows numerous positive cells with a significantly high IgG4/IgG-positive plasma cell ratio. Unlike IgG4-related sialadenitis, infiltrating cells are more monotonous in appearance, with at least occasional foci of atypical lymphocytes being arranged in a sheet pattern. In situ hybridization for light chains is useful for confirming the clonal proliferation of B cells.

6 Lung Disease

Pulmonary involvement in IgG4-RD may take the form of various sizes of lung nodules, lung masses, patchy ground-glass opacities (GGO), infiltrates resembling consolidation, reticular opacities, thickened bronchovascular bundles, central airway stenosis, bronchiectasis, pleural effusion, nodular pleural lesions, and interstitial lung disease (Ryu et al. 2012). However, our knowledge on this organ manifestation is still limited because the collection of a sufficient amount of tissue by transbronchial biopsy remains difficult and some cases are likely to be under-diagnosed. A histological finding that is almost exclusively observed in the lung manifestation is obliterative arteritis, which is characterized by arterial obliteration with sclerosing inflammation (Fig. 4) (Zen et al. 2005, 2009a). In addition,

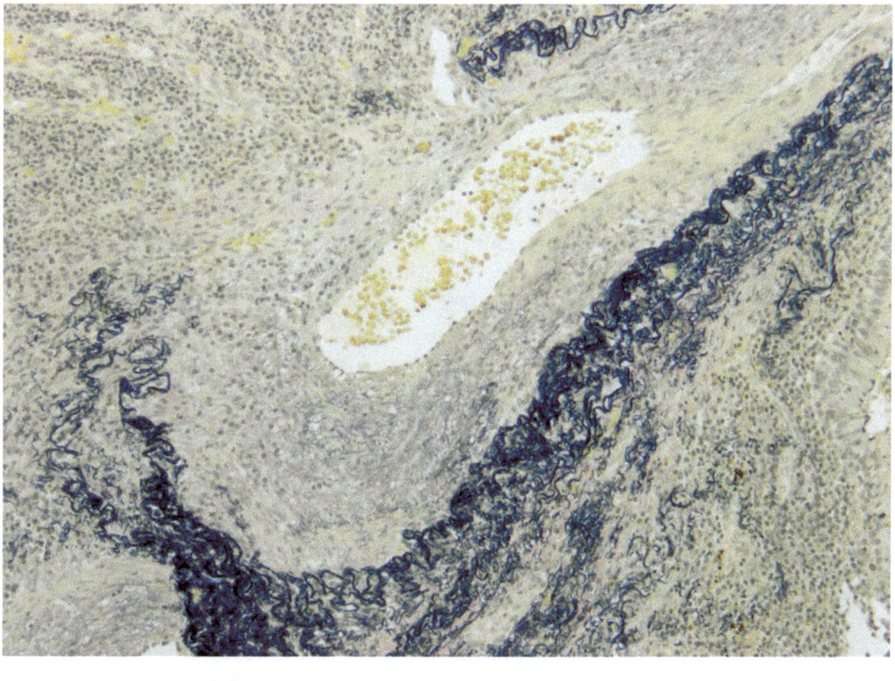

Fig. 4 IgG4-related lung disease. A medium-sized artery is partly obliterated by the inflammatory process (Elastica van Gieson staining)

the characteristic storiform fibrosis observed in pancreatic lesions is less commonly found in pulmonary lesions. A small number of neutrophils may be present in alveolar spaces; therefore, the presence of neutrophils does not exclude the possibility of IgG4-RD at this anatomical site.

A radiopathology correlation study on this organ manifestation revealed that IgG4-related lung disease may be classified into four types on the basis of dominant morphological changes: a solid nodular type exhibiting solitary nodular lesions; a round-shaped GGO type characterized by multiple round-shaped GGO; an alveolar interstitial type mimicking interstitial pneumonia; a bronchovascular type exhibiting thickened interlobular septa and bronchovascular bundles (Inoue et al. 2009). Unlike the other three types, the solid nodular type often exhibits obliterative phlebitis and storiform fibrosis. Obliterative arteritis is also common in this type.

Differential diagnoses of IgG4-related lung disease include multicentric Castleman's disease and granulomatosis with polyangiitis (Chang et al. 2013). Since IgG4-related lung disease and multicentric Castleman's disease share some imaging features, a tissue examination is generally required for this differential diagnosis. Immunostaining for both IgG4 and IgG is particularly important in this aspect because IgG4-positive plasma cells are present in both conditions, but their ratios to IgG-positive plasma cells are typically <40 % in multicentric Castleman's disease. The pattern of fibrosis also differs between the two conditions because hyalinized, densely collagenized fibrosis is commonly observed in multicentric Castleman's disease, but is unusual in IgG4-RD. If the possibility of multicentric Castleman's disease is raised from a pathological aspect, a serological examination of IL-6 concentrations is needed. The measurement of serum IL-6 levels is very useful for this discrimination, but a caveat is that IL-6 is rarely elevated in otherwise typical IgG4-RD.

Patients with granulomatosis with polyangiitis sometimes have elevated serum IgG4 levels. IgG4-positive plasma cells may also be present in tissues with granulomatosis with polyangiitis; therefore, this is a good mimic of IgG4-RD. Although discriminating between these two conditions using biopsy samples may be challenging, the presence of necrosis or vasculitis generally suggests granulomatosis with polyangiitis over IgG4-RD.

7 Periaortitis, Inflammatory Aneurysm, and Retroperitoneal Fibrosis

The abdominal aorta is the most common site of IgG4-related periarteritis. It has traditionally been called retroperitoneal fibrosis (Zen et al. 2006). Since the inflammatory process predominantly affects the adventitia of the aorta, IgG4-related periaortitis appears to be a proper diagnostic term with retroperitoneal fibrosis being applied to sclerosing lesions affecting other anatomical structures in the retroperitoneum (e.g., ureter and broad plaque-like lesions). If the media of the aortic wall is disrupted by the adventitial fibroinflammatory process, the affected aorta shows aneurysmal transformation (Kasashima et al. 2008). Some patients may have IgG4-related periaortitis and retroperitoneal fibrosis. Therefore, IgG4-RD in the retroperitoneum presents with various combinations of periaortitis, aneurysm, and retroperitoneal fibrosis.

Periaortitis and retroperitoneal fibrosis are not always IgG4-related. Approximately 60 % of cases are speculated to have this systemic condition (Zen et al. 2009b; Khosroshahi et al. 2013). Non-IgG4-related sclerosing lesions at these anatomical sites more commonly present with an isolated disease. Similar to IgG4-RD, some cases of non-IgG4-related periaortitis and retroperitoneal fibrosis respond to steroid therapy. Non-IgG4-related cases histologically show less extensive inflammation with a smaller number of IgG4-positive plasma cells than IgG4-RD. However, this differential diagnosis is often difficult based on biopsy samples.

The histology of IgG4-related periaortitis and retroperitoneal fibrosis is basically similar to that in other organs. However, the appearance may be more fibrotic because retroperitoneal IgG4-RD is often asymptomatic and diagnosed at later stages. Long-standing lesions may lack a diffuse inflammatory infiltrate with a smaller number of IgG4-positive cells, thereby making a diagnosis more challenging. The residual changes in vague storiform fibrosis and obliterative phlebitis contribute to a diagnosis of the regressed form of IgG4-related periaortitis (Zen et al. 2012c). Another interesting finding is perineural extension of the inflammatory process, a histological feature particularly common at this anatomical site (Fig. 5). A close clinicopathological correlation (e.g., serum IgG4 concentrations

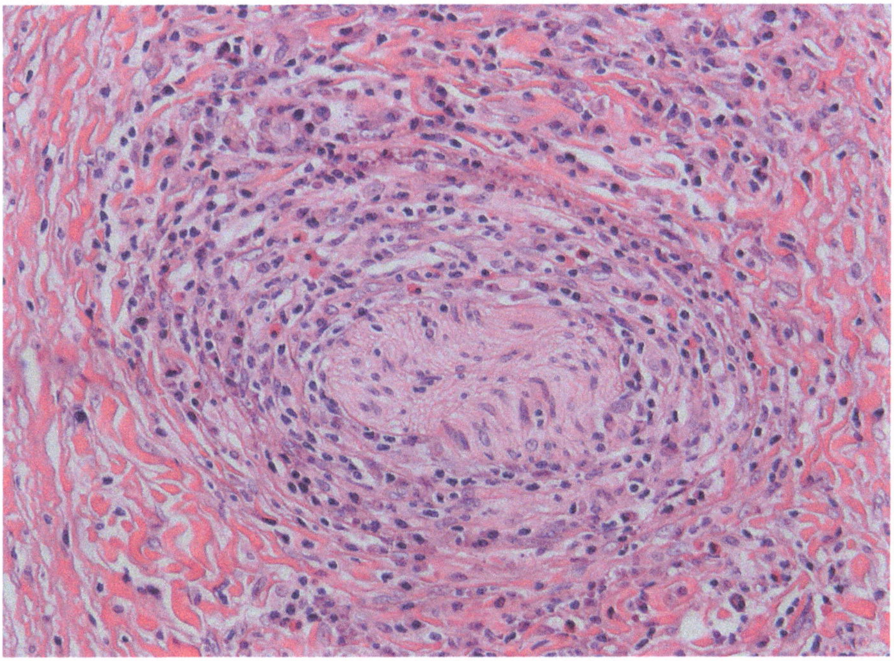

Fig. 5 IgG4-related periaortitis. The inflammatory process shows perineural extension

and other organ involvement) is crucial before establishing a diagnosis in these cases. The disease process mainly affects the adventitia and media, with intimal involvement being less obvious with only mild atherosclerotic changes. This is one reason why IgG4-related periaortitis and arteritis do not cause luminal stenosis and subsequent ischemic injury.

IgG4-related aortic aneurysm differs from infectious aneurysm in that suppurative inflammation is histologically absent and inflammatory serological markers (e.g., C-reactive protein [CRP]) are not elevated. Takayasu arteritis is another differential diagnosis; however, its clinical features (e.g., age and imaging findings) are distinct from those of IgG4-RD. The pathological features of Takayasu arteritis vary with the stage of the disease and include granulomatous inflammation, the degeneration of the elastic layer, adventitial and medial fibrosis, vessel dilatation, and the stenosis or occlusion of involved arteries.

8 Lymphadenopathy

Concomitant regional, rarely generalized, lymphadenopathy is a common feature in patients with IgG4-RD and sometimes appears as the first manifestation of the disease (Cheuk et al. 2008). Several studies have been performed on the morphological and immunohistological findings of IgG4-related lymphadenopathy. These studies demonstrated that lymphadenopathies are histologically distinct from the effects of IgG4-RD in other organs (e.g., storiform fibrosis and obliterative phlebitis are typically absent). Marked histological diversity also complicates the diagnosis, with at least five histological subtypes being identified: Castleman's disease-like morphology (type I), reactive follicular hyperplasia (type II), interfollicular plasmacytosis and immunoblastosis (type III), progressive transformation of germinal center-like disease (type IV), and inflammatory pseudotumor-like disease (type V) (Cheuk and Chan 2012).

Type I disease is characterized by interfollicular expansion with normal to hyperplastic germinal centers penetrated by blood vessels. Abundant plasma cells and scattered eosinophils are apparent in the interfollicular zone (Sato et al. 2009). Type II is morphologically indistinguishable from usual follicular hyperplasia; however, immunostaining confirms the infiltration of IgG4-positive plasma cells. Type III displays marked interfollicular expansion with prominently high endothelial venules, patent sinuses, and atrophic lymphoid follicles. A mixed infiltrate of small lymphocytes, immunoblasts, immature plasma cells, mature plasma cells, and scattered eosinophils has been observed in interfollicular areas. Type IV shows irregular follicular hyperplasia (the so-called progressive transformation of germinal centers) with many interfollicular IgG4-positive plasma cells. Type V is a mass-forming lesion consisting of a lymphoplasmacytic infiltrate and fibrosis, the appearance of which is similar to IgG4-RD in other anatomical sites. These diverse histopathological features potentially represent various immunological reactions occurring in this condition.

However, lymphadenopathy with abundant IgG4-positive plasma cell infiltration may also be detected in multicentric Castleman's disease, rheumatoid arthritis, and other immune-mediated conditions. Owing to these factors, IgG4-related lymphadenopathy cannot be diagnosed on the basis of histological findings alone. Therefore, clinical features and laboratory findings are crucial for these differential diagnoses. Unlike IgG4-RD, multicentric Castleman's disease shows elevated serum levels of CRP, thrombocytosis, anemia, hypoalbuminemia, and hypocholesterolemia. Since IgG4-RD does not affect the synovial membrane, a history of arthritis suggests rheumatoid arthritis over IgG4-RD. Serological rheumatoid factors may be confirmed in either condition; therefore, they are not useful for this discrimination.

9 Summary

Tissue examinations play a key role in the diagnostic process of IgG4-RD. It is important to recognize not only histological features characteristic of this condition, but also microscopic findings that reject the diagnosis. The latter is particularly important to avoid the overdiagnosis of this condition. Although the histology of IgG4-RD is basically similar in any organ manifestation, there are several site-specific changes. A caveat is that IgG4-positive plasma cell infiltration is not entirely specific for IgG4-RD because a large number of studies have suggested that IgG4-positive plasma cells are present in various conditions. Thus, a tissue diagnosis cannot be made based solely on the number of IgG4-positive plasma cells. Immunohistochemical results need to be assessed in combination with H&E findings, and a tissue diagnosis needs to be followed by careful clinicopathological correlations.

References

Chang SY, Keogh KA, Lewis JE, Ryu JH, Cornell LD, Garrity JA, Yi ES (2013) IgG4-positive plasma cells in granulomatosis with polyangiitis (Wegener's): a clinicopathologic and immunohistochemical study on 43 granulomatosis with polyangiitis and 20 control cases. Hum Pathol 44(11):2432–2437. doi:10.1016/j.humpath.2013.05.023

Cheuk W, Chan JK (2012) Lymphadenopathy of IgG4-related disease: an underdiagnosed and overdiagnosed entity. Semin Diagn Pathol 29(4):226–234. doi:10.1053/j.semdp.2012.07.001

Cheuk W, Yuen HK, Chu SY, Chiu EK, Lam LK, Chan JK (2008) Lymphadenopathy of IgG4-related sclerosing disease. Am J Surg Pathol 32(5):671–681. doi:10.1097/PAS.0b013e318157c068

Deshpande V, Sainani NI, Chung RT, Pratt DS, Mentha G, Rubbia-Brandt L, Lauwers GY (2009) IgG4-associated cholangitis: a comparative histological and immunophenotypic study with primary sclerosing cholangitis on liver biopsy material. Mod Pathol 22(10):1287–1295. doi:10.1038/modpathol.2009.94

Deshpande V, Zen Y, Chan JK, Yi EE, Sato Y, Yoshino T, Kloppel G, Heathcote JG, Khosroshahi A, Ferry JA, Aalberse RC, Bloch DB, Brugge WR, Bateman AC, Carruthers MN, Chari ST, Cheuk W, Cornell LD, Fernandez-Del Castillo C, Forcione DG, Hamilos DL, Kamisawa T, Kasashima S, Kawa S, Kawano M, Lauwers GY, Masaki Y, Nakanuma Y, Notohara K, Okazaki K, Ryu JK, Saeki T, Sahani DV, Smyrk TC, Stone JR, Takahira M, Webster GJ, Yamamoto M, Zamboni G, Umehara H, Stone JH (2012) Consensus statement on the pathology of IgG4-related disease. Mod Pathol 25(9):1181–1192. doi:10.1038/modpathol.2012.72

Hamano H, Kawa S, Horiuchi A, Unno H, Furuya N, Akamatsu T, Fukushima M, Nikaido T, Nakayama K, Usuda N, Kiyosawa K (2001) High serum IgG4 concentrations in patients with sclerosing pancreatitis. N Engl J Med 344(10):732–738. doi:10.1056/nejm200103083441005

Hamano H, Kawa S, Ochi Y, Unno H, Shiba N, Wajiki M, Nakazawa K, Shimojo H, Kiyosawa K (2002) Hydronephrosis associated with retroperitoneal fibrosis and sclerosing pancreatitis. Lancet 359(9315):1403–1404

Hart PA, Zen Y, Chari ST (2015) Recent advances in autoimmune pancreatitis. Gastroenterology 149(1):39–51. doi:10.1053/j.gastro.2015.03.010

Inoue D, Zen Y, Abo H, Gabata T, Demachi H, Kobayashi T, Yoshikawa J, Miyayama S, Yasui M, Nakanuma Y, Matsui O (2009) Immunoglobulin G4-related lung disease: CT findings with pathologic correlations. Radiology 251(1):260–270. doi:10.1148/radiol.2511080965

Inoue D, Yoshida K, Yoneda N, Ozaki K, Matsubara T, Nagai K, Okumura K, Toshima F, Toyama J, Minami T, Matsui O, Gabata T, Zen Y (2015) IgG4-related disease: dataset of 235 consecutive patients. Medicine 94(15):e680. doi:10.1097/md.0000000000000680

Kamisawa T, Zen Y, Pillai S, Stone JH (2014) IgG4-related disease. Lancet. doi:10.1016/S0140-6736(14)60720-0

Kasashima S, Zen Y, Kawashima A, Konishi K, Sasaki H, Endo M, Matsumoto Y, Kawakami K, Kasashima F, Moriya M, Kimura K, Ohtake H, Nakanuma Y (2008) Inflammatory abdominal aortic aneurysm: close relationship to IgG4-related periaortitis. Am J Surg Pathol 32(2):197–204. doi:10.1097/PAS.0b013e3181342f0d

Khosroshahi A, Carruthers MN, Stone JH, Shinagare S, Sainani N, Hasserjian RP, Deshpande V (2013) Rethinking Ormond's disease: "idiopathic" retroperitoneal fibrosis in the era of IgG4-related disease. Medicine 92(2):82–91. doi:10.1097/MD.0b013e318289610f

Kitagawa S, Zen Y, Harada K, Sasaki M, Sato Y, Minato H, Watanabe K, Kurumaya H, Katayanagi K, Masuda S, Niwa H, Tsuneyama K, Saito K, Haratake J, Takagawa K, Nakanuma Y (2005) Abundant IgG4-positive plasma cell infiltration characterizes chronic sclerosing sialadenitis (Kuttner's tumor). Am J Surg Pathol 29(6):783–791

Notohara K, Burgart LJ, Yadav D, Chari S, Smyrk TC (2003) Idiopathic chronic pancreatitis with periductal lymphoplasmacytic infiltration: clinicopathologic features of 35 cases. Am J Surg Pathol 27(8):1119–1127

Okazaki K, Uchida K (2015) Autoimmune pancreatitis: the past, present, and future. Pancreas 44(7):1006–1016. doi:10.1097/mpa.0000000000000382

Ryu JH, Sekiguchi H, Yi ES (2012) Pulmonary manifestations of immunoglobulin G4-related sclerosing disease. Eur Respir J 39(1):180–186. doi:10.1183/09031936.00025211

Sato Y, Takata K, Ichimura K, Tanaka T, Morito T, Tamura M, Yoshino T (2008) IgG4-producing marginal zone B-cell lymphoma. Int J Hematol 88(4):428–433. doi:10.1007/s12185-008-0170-8

Sato Y, Kojima M, Takata K, Morito T, Asaoku H, Takeuchi T, Mizobuchi K, Fujihara M, Kuraoka K, Nakai T, Ichimura K, Tanaka T, Tamura M, Nishikawa Y, Yoshino T (2009) Systemic IgG4-related lymphadenopathy: a clinical and pathologic comparison to multicentric Castleman's disease. Mod Pathol 22(4):589–599. doi:10.1038/modpathol.2009.17

Shimosegawa T, Chari ST, Frulloni L, Kamisawa T, Kawa S, Mino-Kenudson M, Kim MH, Kloppel G, Lerch MM, Lohr M, Notohara K, Okazaki K, Schneider A, Zhang L (2011) International consensus diagnostic criteria for autoimmune pancreatitis: guidelines of the

International Association of Pancreatology. Pancreas 40(3):352–358. doi:10.1097/MPA.0b013e3182142fd2
Stone JH, Zen Y, Deshpande V (2012) IgG4-related disease. N Engl J Med 366(6):539–551. doi:10.1056/NEJMra1104650
Umemura T, Zen Y, Hamano H, Kawa S, Nakanuma Y, Kiyosawa K (2007) Immunoglobin G4-hepatopathy: association of immunoglobin G4-bearing plasma cells in liver with autoimmune pancreatitis. Hepatology 46(2):463–471. doi:10.1002/hep.21700
Yamamoto M, Harada S, Ohara M, Suzuki C, Naishiro Y, Yamamoto H, Takahashi H, Imai K (2005) Clinical and pathological differences between Mikulicz's disease and Sjogren's syndrome. Rheumatology (Oxford, England) 44(2):227–234. doi:10.1093/rheumatology/keh447
Zamboni G, Luttges J, Capelli P, Frulloni L, Cavallini G, Pederzoli P, Leins A, Longnecker D, Kloppel G (2004) Histopathological features of diagnostic and clinical relevance in autoimmune pancreatitis: a study on 53 resection specimens and 9 biopsy specimens. Virchows Archiv 445(6):552–563. doi:10.1007/s00428-004-1140-z
Zen Y, Nakanuma Y (2010) IgG4-related disease: a cross-sectional study of 114 cases. Am J Surg Pathol 34(12):1812–1819. doi:10.1097/PAS.0b013e3181f7266b
Zen Y, Harada K, Sasaki M, Sato Y, Tsuneyama K, Haratake J, Kurumaya H, Katayanagi K, Masuda S, Niwa H, Morimoto H, Miwa A, Uchiyama A, Portmann BC, Nakanuma Y (2004) IgG4-related sclerosing cholangitis with and without hepatic inflammatory pseudotumor, and sclerosing pancreatitis-associated sclerosing cholangitis: do they belong to a spectrum of sclerosing pancreatitis? Am J Surg Pathol 28(9):1193–1203
Zen Y, Kitagawa S, Minato H, Kurumaya H, Katayanagi K, Masuda S, Niwa H, Fujimura M, Nakanuma Y (2005) IgG4-positive plasma cells in inflammatory pseudotumor (plasma cell granuloma) of the lung. Hum Pathol 36(7):710–717. doi:10.1016/j.humpath.2005.05.011
Zen Y, Sawazaki A, Miyayama S, Notsumata K, Tanaka N, Nakanuma Y (2006) A case of retroperitoneal and mediastinal fibrosis exhibiting elevated levels of IgG4 in the absence of sclerosing pancreatitis (autoimmune pancreatitis). Hum Pathol 37(2):239–243. doi:10.1016/j.humpath.2005.11.001
Zen Y, Fujii T, Sato Y, Masuda S, Nakanuma Y (2007) Pathological classification of hepatic inflammatory pseudotumor with respect to IgG4-related disease. Mod Pathol 20(8):884–894. doi:10.1038/modpathol.3800836
Zen Y, Inoue D, Kitao A, Onodera M, Abo H, Miyayama S, Gabata T, Matsui O, Nakanuma Y (2009a) IgG4-related lung and pleural disease: a clinicopathologic study of 21 cases. Am J Surg Pathol 33(12):1886–1893. doi:10.1097/PAS.0b013e3181bd535b
Zen Y, Onodera M, Inoue D, Kitao A, Matsui O, Nohara T, Namiki M, Kasashima S, Kawashima A, Matsumoto Y, Katayanagi K, Murata T, Ishizawa S, Hosaka N, Kuriki K, Nakanuma Y (2009b) Retroperitoneal fibrosis: a clinicopathologic study with respect to immunoglobulin G4. Am J Surg Pathol 33(12):1833–1839
Zen Y, Grammatikopoulos T, Heneghan MA, Vergani D, Mieli-Vergani G, Portmann BC (2012a) Sclerosing cholangitis with granulocytic epithelial lesion: a benign form of sclerosing cholangiopathy. Am J Surg Pathol 36(10):1555–1561. doi:10.1097/PAS.0b013e31825faae0
Zen Y, Ishikawa A, Ogiso S, Heaton N, Portmann B (2012b) Follicular cholangitis and pancreatitis—clinicopathological features and differential diagnosis of an under-recognized entity. Histopathology 60(2):261–269. doi:10.1111/j.1365-2559.2011.04078.x
Zen Y, Kasashima S, Inoue D (2012c) Retroperitoneal and aortic manifestations of immunoglobulin G4-related disease. Semin Diagn Pathol 29(4):212–218. doi:10.1053/j.semdp.2012.07.003
Zen Y, Nakanuma Y, Portmann B (2012d) Immunoglobulin G4-related sclerosing cholangitis: pathologic features and histologic mimics. Semin Diagn Pathol 29(4):205–211. doi:10.1053/j.semdp.2012.07.005
Zen Y, Britton D, Mitra V, Pike I, Heaton N, Quaglia A (2015) A global proteomic study identifies distinct pathological features of IgG4-related and primary sclerosing cholangitis. Histopathology. doi:10.1111/his.12813

Zen Y, Kawakami H, Kim JH (2016) IgG4-related sclerosing cholangitis: all we need to know. J Gastroenterol. doi:10.1007/s00535-016-1163-7

Zhang L, Chari S, Smyrk TC, Deshpande V, Kloppel G, Kojima M, Liu X, Longnecker DS, Mino-Kenudson M, Notohara K, Rodriguez-Justo M, Srivastava A, Zamboni G, Zen Y (2011) Autoimmune pancreatitis (AIP) type 1 and type 2: an international consensus study on histopathologic diagnostic criteria. Pancreas 40(8):1172–1179. doi:10.1097/MPA.0b013e318233bec5

The Immunobiology of Immunoglobulin G4 and Complement Activation Pathways in IgG4-Related Disease

Shigeyuki Kawa

Abstract High serum immunoglobulin (Ig) G4 concentration and abundant IgG4-bearing plasma cell infiltration are characteristic features in autoimmune pancreatitis (AIP). AIP is also complicated with a variety of other organ involvements that commonly share marked IgG4-bearing plasma cell infiltration, suggesting the existence of a systemic disease associated with IgG4 currently recognized as IgG4-related disease (IgG4-RD). However, it is controversial whether IgG4 plays a role in the pathogenesis of AIP or IgG4-RD through such characteristic attributes as Fab-arm exchange and rheumatoid factor (RF)-like activity. Hypocomplementemia has been observed in AIP and several other IgG4-RDs. Muraki et al. reported that complements C3 and C4 were decreased in 36 % of patients with AIP, which implicated the complement activation system in disease pathogenesis. AIP patients with a high level of immune complexes showed serum elevation of IgG4-type immune complexes in an active disease stage, elevated serum IgG1 concentration, and decreased C3 and C4 values. This inferred that while IgG4 may have had little contribution to complement activation, IgG1 played a prominent role via the classical pathway. On the other hand, Sugimoto et al. observed that polyethylene glycol-precipitated immune complexes from patients with IgG4-RD and hypocomplementemia had the ability to activate the complement system through both the classical and the mannose-binding lectin pathways and that IgG4 might participate in the complement activation system. Thus, debate continues on which complement activation systems are working in AIP and IgG4-RD and whether they are associated with the pathogenesis of these conditions.

S. Kawa (✉)
Center for Health, Safety and Environmental Management,
Shinshu University, Matsumoto, Japan
e-mail: skawapc@shinshu-u.ac.jp

Current Topics in Microbiology and Immunology (2017) 401: 61–74
DOI 10.1007/82_2016_39

Published Online: 16 September 2016

Contents

1 The Immunobiology of Immunoglobulin G4 (IgG4)

1.1 Recognized Functions of IgG4

We first reported in 2001 that high serum IgG4 concentrations were found frequently and specifically in patients with autoimmune pancreatitis (AIP) (Hamano et al. 2001). Later, in 2002, we described how abundant IgG4-bearing plasma cell infiltration was recognized both in affected pancreatic tissues of AIP and in extra-pancreatic lesions (Hamano et al. 2002). AIP is also complicated with a variety of other organ involvements that commonly share the feature of marked IgG4-bearing plasma cell infiltration (Hamano et al. 2002), suggesting the presence of a systemic disease associated with IgG4 now recognized as IgG4-related disease (IgG4-RD). Although the concept of IgG4-RD has become widely accepted (Stone et al. 2012), the precise role of IgG4 in the pathogenesis of AIP and IgG4-RD remains unclear.

The human IgG is composed of 4 subclasses, IgG1-4, whose classification and nomenclature reflect the order of their discovery and amount and ratio in the serum. Accordingly, IgG1 was discovered first as the major component of IgG, while IgG4 was the lastly identified and most minor IgG constituent. Although mouse IgG also has subclasses, its naming is based on electrophoretic mobility, meaning that mouse IgG1 does not necessarily correspond to human IgG1, but rather functionally to human IgG4 (Aalberse et al. 2009). Thus, the study of mouse IgG1 may provide insights on the function of its human counterpart.

The primary roles of IgG4 appear to be divided into blocking antibody and disease pathogenesis, by which the former contributes to the attenuation of allergic reactions (Aalberse 2011) and the latter factors in the pathogenesis of certain diseases, such as pemphigus vulgaris (Rock et al. 1989), idiopathic membranous glomerulonephritis (Beck et al. 2009), acquired thrombocytopenic purpura (Ferrari et al. 2009), and muscle-specific kinase myasthenia gravis (Plomp et al. 2012). The allergen-specific IgG4 antibodies used in immunotherapy were originally considered to bind circulating allergic substances and inhibit binding to IgE antibodies on mast cells to thereby block cell activation in allergic reactions. However, their major role is now believed to inhibit the correlations between allergens and IgE antibodies, which then attenuates the inflammatory action of Th2 cells (Aalberse 2011).

On the other hand, in patients with pemphigus vulgaris, the IgG4-type autoantibody-to-cell adhesion molecule desmoglein possibly functions as a pathogenic antibody that produces bullous skin lesions (Rock et al. 1989). Pemphigus vulgaris is closely associated with *HLA DRB1*04:02*, which suggests that this gene product on antigen-presenting cells presents a degradation peptide of desmoglein to T cells (Wucherpfennig et al. 1995), resulting in the production of antigen-specific IgG4 autoantibodies. In fact, subcutaneous injection of purified desmoglein-specific IgG4 antibodies from collected patient serum causes the formation of pemphigus-like bullous lesions in neonatal mice (Shirakata et al. 1990). Similar to pemphigus vulgaris, IgG4-type pathogenic autoantibodies were reported to correspond to ADAMST13 in acquired thrombocytopenic purpura (Ferrari et al. 2009) and membrane-type phospholipase 2 receptor in idiopathic membranous glomerulonephritis (Beck et al. 2009; Yang et al. 2016). However, it remains uncertain whether IgG4-type pathogenic antibodies exert a role in AIP.

Recently, Shiokawa et al. demonstrated that subcutaneous injection of IgG from AIP patients, but not control IgG, caused pancreatic and salivary injury in neonatal mice (Shiokawa et al. 2016). Although pancreatic injury was also induced by patient IgG1 or IgG4, the potent pathogenic activity of IgG1 was significantly inhibited by simultaneous injection of IgG4. These results suggested that circulating IgG4 in AIP patients may have both pathogenic and protective roles. Immunostaining of the IgG subtypes disclosed that IgG4 recognizing autoantigens in the extracellular space competed with IgG1 targeting the same antigens and that the binding of pathogenic IgG1 to target antigens was inhibited by the higher binding activity of IgG4. They speculated that the autoantibodies in AIP serum recognized molecules involved in cell–ECM adhesion (Shiokawa et al. 2016).

1.2 Association between AIP and IgG4

The characteristic feature in electrophoresis of AIP patient serum is known as β-γ bridging, which sparked the discovery of a close association between AIP and IgG4 (Hamano et al. 2001). β-γ bridging represents a smooth transition from the β peak to the γ one, which was later found to be caused by high serum IgG4 concentrations by the immune-fixation method (Fig. 1). Of the 4 human IgG subclasses, IgG4 represents the smallest fraction at only 4–6 %. We earlier examined whether IgG4 was increased in patients with AIP by comparing the serum concentrations of each IgG subclass between 20 AIP subjects and 20 age- and sex-matched controls and found that the IgG4 values in AIP serum were over 10 times higher than those in controls, while the values of other subclasses were comparable (Hamano et al. 2001). We then sought to determine whether serum IgG4 elevation was specific to

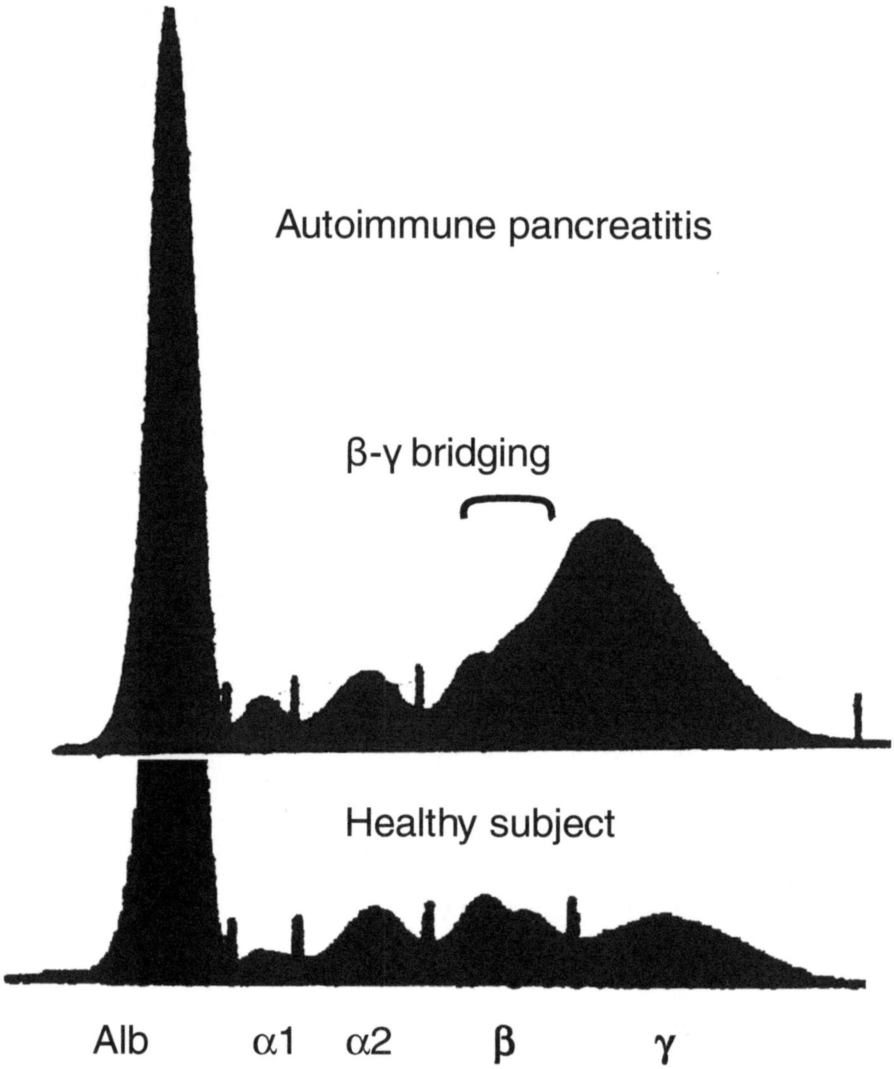

Fig. 1 Paper electrophoresis of serum in AIP reveals β-γ globulin bridging (from Tan to Sui 22;603–608:2001 in a Japanese publication. Reprinted with permission from Igakutosho-shuppan, Ltd.)

AIP by comparing the serum IgG4 concentrations of various conditions, including pancreatic cancer, ordinary chronic pancreatitis, primary biliary cirrhosis, primary sclerosing cholangitis, Sjögren's syndrome, and normal subjects and discovered that serum IgG4 was elevated in over 90 % of AIP patients but scarcely in other diseases (Fig. 2) (Hamano et al. 2001). AIP shows clinical and imaging findings similar to those of pancreatic cancer; previous reports showed that 2–3 % of

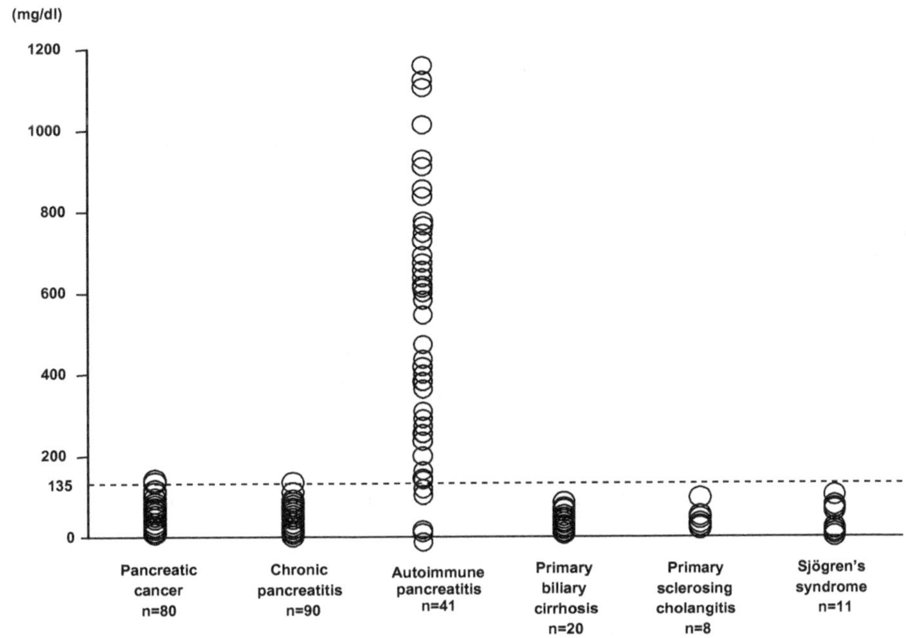

Fig. 2 Scattergram of serum IgG4 values in various conditions, including AIP (from Hamano et al. (2001), Copyright (c) 2001 Massachusetts Medical Society. Reprinted with permission)

pancreatic tissues that had been resected based on a diagnosis of pancreatic cancer were later rediagnosed as lymphoplasmacytic sclerosing pancreatitis corresponding to the histology of AIP (Kawaguchi et al. 1991; Abraham et al. 2003). As AIP responds well to corticosteroid treatment, correct diagnosis is urgent and useless surgery should be avoided. We later evaluated the diagnostic utility of IgG4 in the differentiation of AIP from pancreatic cancer and uncovered the favorable results of 97 % accuracy, 95 % sensitivity, and 97 % specificity (Hamano et al. 2001). These results indicated that serum IgG4 assaying was useful not only for the diagnosis of AIP, but also for its differentiation from pancreatic cancer. Furthermore, serum IgG4 values decreased dramatically after corticosteroid treatment and increased again during relapse, thus representing a sensitive marker of disease activity, and could predict AIP relapse effectively even in the subclinical phase (Kawa and Hamano 2007).

1.3 Establishment of the New Disease Concept IgG4-RD

We previously confirmed abundant IgG4-bearing plasma cell infiltration in 3 tissues of retroperitoneal fibrosis in addition to that of complicating AIP (Hamano et al.

2002). These findings suggested that IgG4-bearing plasma cell infiltration in other organ involvement could help in the diagnosis of AIP and moreover indicated the presence of a systemic disease associated with IgG4. Following this report, many investigators have proposed new systemic disease concepts associated with IgG4 (Kamisawa et al. 2004; Yamamoto et al. 2006; Masaki et al. 2008), which have culminated in the establishment of the disease concept IgG4-RD in Japan (Umehara et al. 2011). IgG4-RD has since been widely adopted worldwide after an international symposium on IgG4-RD in 2013 in Boston (Stone et al. 2012).

1.4 Peculiar Characteristics of IgG4: Fab-Arm Exchange and Rheumatoid Factor (RF)-Like Activity

IgG4 may contribute to the pathogenesis of AIP and IgG4-RD based on its peculiar characteristics, namely Fab-arm exchange (van der Neut et al. 2007) and RF-like activity (Kawa et al. 2008).

1.4.1 Fab-Arm Exchange

Previous reports have shown that IgG4 lacks the cross-linking activity to bind soluble antigens to those in a solid-phase, representing a non-precipitating or monovalent antibody (van der Zee et al. 1986). IgG4 possesses a loose connection at the disulfide bond of H chains, which easily causes the dissociation of original half molecules and the association of new half molecules from neighboring IgG4 to result in different antigen reactivity for each Fab in the same IgG4 antibody, i.e., Fab-arm exchange (Fig. 3) (van der Neut et al. 2007; Rispens 2011). Fab-arm exchange precludes same antigen cross-linking and leads to the formation non-precipitating antibody immune complexes. Thus, the lack of cross-linking activity of IgG4 is due to its hetero-bivalence, which may be related to its roles in anti-inflammation (Aalberse et al. 2009).

1.4.2 RF-Like Activity (Novel RF)

IgG4 has also been reported to have RF activity, that is, binding to the Fc portion of IgG (Hennig et al. 2000; Mukai et al. 2004). We confirmed that IgG4 from AIP serum bound to IgG1, IgG2, IgG3, and IgG4 from myeloma proteins, as well as to IgG Fc, which represented RF activity (Fig. 4). However, IgG4 Fc, but not IgG4 Fab, bound to IgG Fc, indicating that this phenomenon was via Fc-Fc interactions

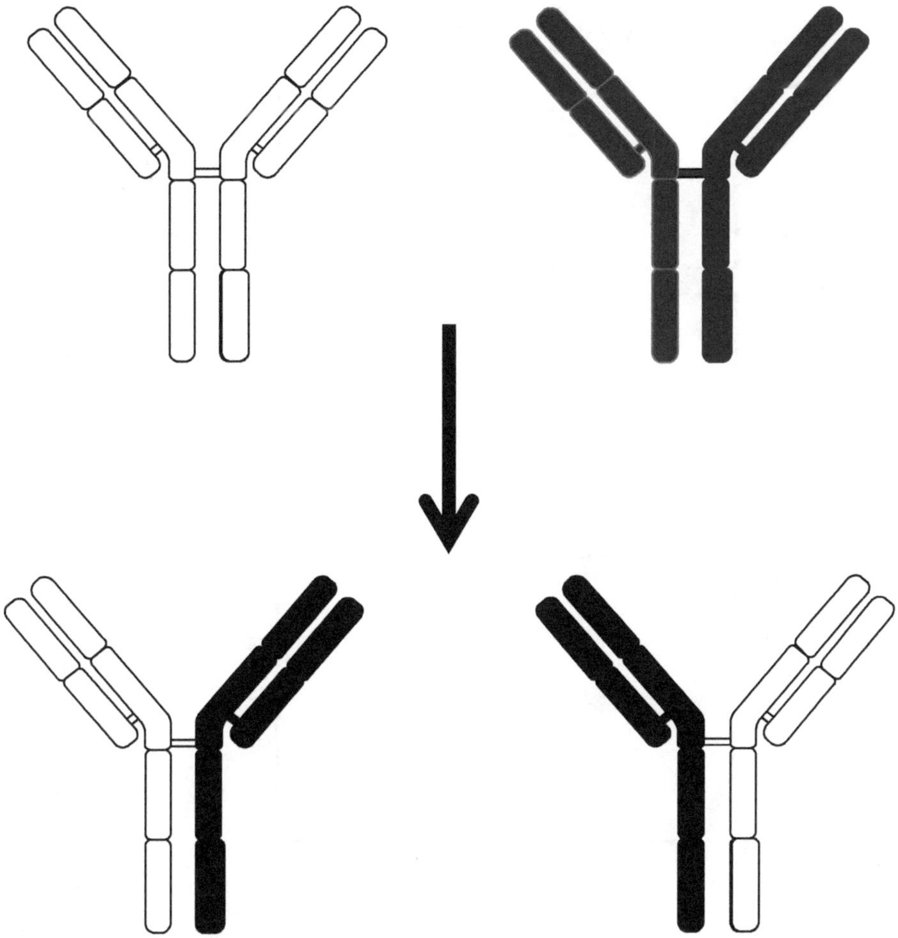

Fig. 3 Fab-arm exchange, a characteristic feature of IgG4

and not the typical Fab-Fc interactions of RF activity (Fig. 5), for which we have defined as novel RF (Fig. 6) (Kawa et al. 2008). Furthermore, human IgG4 was seen to bind to the Fc portions of various animal IgGs (Ito et al. 2010). Although the exact role of this IgG4 novel RF-like activity remains unclear, it may act as a step in the process of IgG4 Fab-arm exchange. Different IgG4 molecules with the same antigen reactivity may associate via Fc-Fc interaction and then exchange half molecules of each IgG4, resulting in Fab-arm exchange with different epitope reactivity (Rispens 2009).

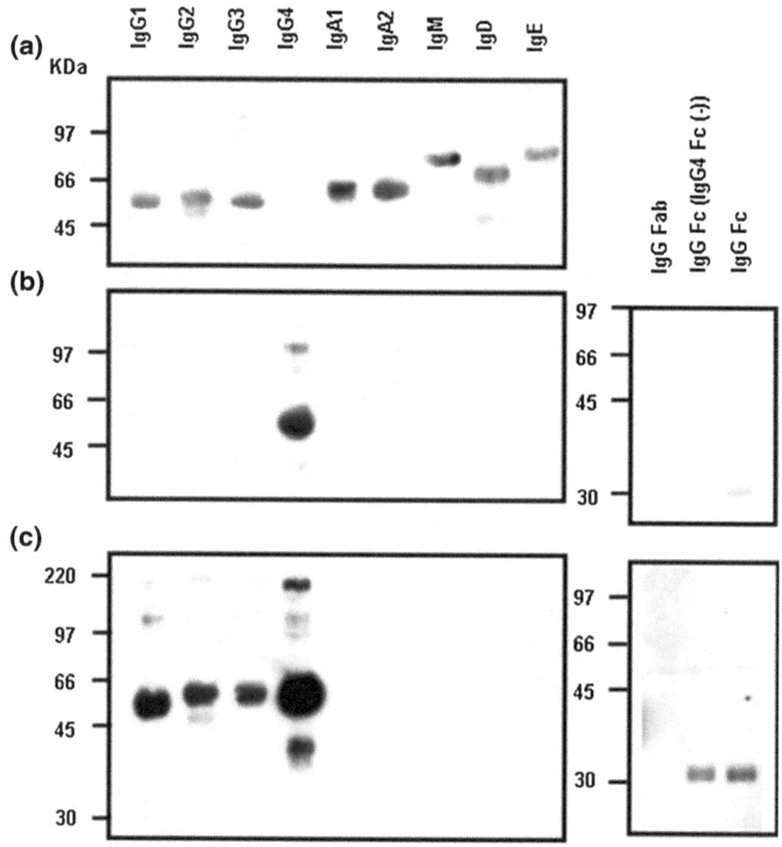

Fig. 4 Reactivity of human IgG4 to various immunoglobulin classes and subclasses. Western blot analysis demonstrates the reactivity of IgG4 in the pooled serum of patients with AIP to various human immunoglobulin subclasses. **a** The identity of each commercially purchased immunoglobulin myeloma protein is confirmed upon reaction with the corresponding HRP-labeled anti-isotype antibodies: IgG1κ, IgG2κ, IgG3κ, IgA1κ, IgA2κ, IgMκ, IgDκ, and IgEλ. **b** Similarly, HRP-labeled antibodies against IgG4 Fc specifically react to IgG4κ and IgG Fc (faint band in the right panel), but not to IgG Fab or Ig Fc lacking IgG4 Fc. **c** An identical membrane to panel A was first subjected to pooled AIP serum and then to HRP-labeled anti-IgG4 Fc antibody which, in contrast to panel B, reacts to IgG1κ, IgG2κ, IgG3κ, IgG Fc, and affinity-purified IgG Fc lacking IgG4 Fc, but not to other human immunoglobulins or IgG Fab, establishing that AIP patient IgG4 reacts to IgG1, 2, and 3 Fc [from Kawa et al. (2008)]

2 Complement Activation Pathways in IgG4-RD

2.1 AIP and the Complement Activation System

The complement activation system is composed of 3 pathways: the classical pathway, the alternative pathway, and the mannose-binding lectin (MBL) pathway.

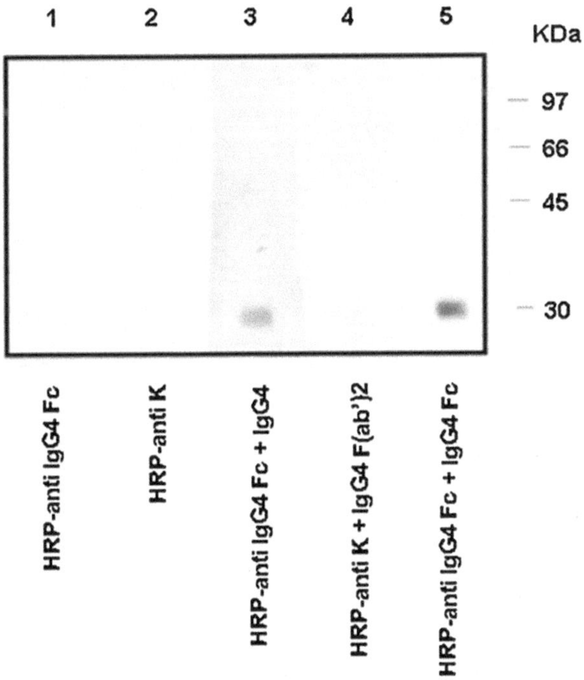

Fig. 5 Topology of IgG4-IgG interactions. Western blotting is used to establish whether the Fc or Fab portion(s) of IgG4 react to IgG Fc. IgG Fc lacking IgG4 Fc was blotted in each lane. HRP-labeled anti-human IgG4 Fc or HRP-labeled anti-human κ light chain shows no reactivity to IgG Fc lacking IgG4 Fc (lanes 1 and 2). HRP-labeled anti-IgG4 Fc antibody reacts in lanes 3 and 5 previously incubated with purified IgG4 and IgG4 Fc, respectively. HRP-labeled anti-human κ light chain has no reactivity in lane 4, which has been incubated with IgG4 F(ab')2. These results indicate that IgG4 binds to IgG Fc by its own Fc, and not its Fab as in classical RF [from Kawa et al. (2008)]

Muraki et al. reported that complements C3 and C4 were decreased in 36 % of patients with AIP, which suggested that the complement activation system factored in disease pathogenesis (Muraki et al. 2006). In AIP, decreased C4 negates the contribution of the alternative pathway. The MBL pathway is a member of the innate immune system that functions as a defensive mechanism against microbial or viral infections (Medzhitov and Janeway 2000). On the other hand, this pathway has been implicated in the development of various conditions, including systemic lupus erythematosus, rheumatoid arthritis, Crohn's disease, and ulcerative colitis. If the MBL pathway indeed contributed to the pathogenesis of AIP, it would be presumable that serum MBL concentrations in AIP patients were lower than those of controls and chronic pancreatitis patients. However, we found that MBL levels in AIP were higher than those in other conditions, detected no differences in values before and after corticosteroid treatment, and observed no association with disease activity, implying that the MBL pathway did not contribute to AIP pathogenesis.

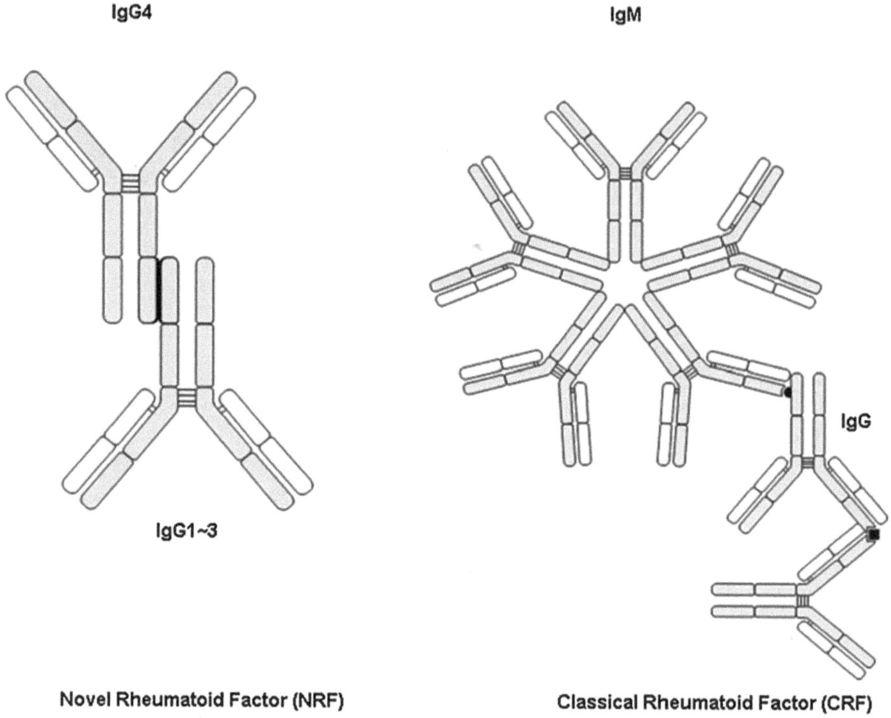

Fig. 6 Novel RF. Schematic representation of 2 distinct modes of Ig-Ig interactions. On the left, IgG4 Fc interacts with Ig Fc. On the right, IgM RF recognizes IgG in a classical Fab-Fc recognition pattern [from Kawa et al. (2008)]

Furthermore, patients with AIP showed serum elevation of IgG4-type immune complexes in an active disease state. By comparing various parameters between an AIP patient group with high serum immune complex levels as determined by C1q assays and one with low levels, we uncovered a significantly higher serum IgG1 concentration and decreased C4 and C3 values in the higher immune complex group (Muraki et al. 2006). Since IgG4 did not bind to C1q, it appeared to have no contribution to complement activation, while IgG1 seemed strongly implicated via the classical pathway.

2.2 IgG4-RD and the Complement Activation System

Apart from AIP, hypocomplementemia has been observed in other IgG4-RDs, especially IgG4-related kidney disease (Saeki et al. 2010). Saeki et al. identified 6 patients with high serum IgG4 levels among 10 patients with hypocomplementemia of unknown etiology (Saeki et al. 2009). Sugimoto et al. investigated which IgG subclasses contributed to the activation of the complement pathway in IgG4-RD patients with hypocomplementemia (Sugimoto et al. 2016) and noted reduced complement activity in all pathways in the sera of affected patients. Although the serum levels of C1q-binding IgG4 were elevated in IgG4-RD patients with hypocomplementemia, they were considered to be attributable to circulating immune complexes (ICs), which was confirmed by analyzing the IgG subclass composition of polyethylene glycol-precipitated ICs (PEG-ICs). PEG-ICs from IgG4-RD patients with hypocomplementemia showed a marked reduction in CH50 and reduced complement activity in the classical and MBL pathways. These results suggested that PEG-ICs from patients with IgG4-RD and hypocomplementemia had the ability to activate the complement system through multiple pathways and that IgG4 might participate in complement activation (Sugimoto et al. 2016). These findings appear to be contrary to the previously accepted theory and the results of Muraki's study.

The discrepancies between the results of Muraki's investigation and those of Sugimoto may be attributed to the difference in methods applied by the studies, in which the former was an indirect observation, while the latter was a direct one, or to the varying diseases analyzed, which were AIP and mainly Mikulicz's disease, respectively (Sugimoto et al. 2016). Thus, there is a controversy on what complement activation systems are working in AIP and IgG4-RD and whether they are associated with the pathogenesis of these diseases.

References

Aalberse R (2011) The role of IgG antibodies in allergy and immunotherapy. Allergy 66(Suppl 95):28–30. doi:10.1111/j.1398-9995.2011.02628.x

Aalberse RC, Stapel SO, Schuurman J, Rispens T (2009) Immunoglobulin G4: an odd antibody. Clin Exp Allergy 39(4):469–477. doi:10.1111/j.1365-2222.2009.03207.x (CEA3207 [pii])

Abraham SC, Cruz-Correa M, Argani P, Furth EE, Hruban RH, Boitnott JK (2003) Lymphoplasmacytic chronic cholecystitis and biliary tract disease in patients with lymphoplasmacytic sclerosing pancreatitis. Am J Surg Pathol 27(4):441–451

Beck LH Jr, Bonegio RG, Lambeau G, Beck DM, Powell DW, Cummins TD et al (2009) M-type phospholipase A2 receptor as target antigen in idiopathic membranous nephropathy. N Engl J Med 361(1):11–21. doi:10.1056/NEJMoa0810457 (361/1/11 [pii])

Ferrari S, Mudde GC, Rieger M, Veyradier A, Kremer Hovinga JA, Scheiflinger F (2009) IgG subclass distribution of anti-ADAMTS13 antibodies in patients with acquired thrombotic thrombocytopenic purpura. Journal of thrombosis and haemostasis: JTH. 7(10):1703–1710. doi:10.1111/j.1538-7836.2009.03568.x

Hamano H, Kawa S, Horiuchi A, Unno H, Furuya N, Akamatsu T et al (2001) High serum IgG4 concentrations in patients with sclerosing pancreatitis. New Engl J Med 344(10):732–738

Hamano H, Kawa S, Ochi Y, Unno H, Shiba N, Wajiki M et al (2002) Hydronephrosis associated with retroperitoneal fibrosis and sclerosing pancreatitis. Lancet 359(9315):1403–1404. doi:10.1016/S0140-6736(02)08359-9

Hennig C, Rink L, Kirchner H (2000) Evidence for presence of IgG4 anti-immunoglobulin autoantibodies in all human beings. Lancet 355(9215):1617–1618. doi:10.1016/S0140-6736(00)02223-6

Ito T, Kitahara K, Umemura T, Ota M, Shimozuru Y, Kawa S et al (2010) A novel heterophilic antibody interaction involves IgG4. Scand J Immunol 71(2):109–114. doi:10.1111/j.1365-3083.2009.02353.x (SJI2353 [pii])

Kamisawa T, Funata N, Hayashi Y (2004) Lymphoplasmacytic sclerosing pancreatitis is a pancreatic lesion of IgG4-related systemic disease. Am J Surg Pathol. 28(8):1114. doi:00000478-200408000-00023 [pii]

Kawa S, Hamano H (2007) Clinical features of autoimmune pancreatitis. J Gastroenterol 42(Suppl 18):9–14. doi:10.1007/s00535-007-2044-x

Kawa S, Kitahara K, Hamano H, Ozaki Y, Arakura N, Yoshizawa K et al (2008) A novel immunoglobulin-immunoglobulin interaction in autoimmunity. PLoS ONE 3(2):e1637. doi:10.1371/journal.pone.0001637

Kawaguchi K, Koike M, Tsuruta K, Okamoto A, Tabata I, Fujita N (1991) Lymphoplasmacytic sclerosing pancreatitis with cholangitis: a variant of primary sclerosing cholangitis extensively involving pancreas. Hum Pathol 22(4):387–395

Masaki Y, Dong L, Kurose N, Kitagawa K, Morikawa Y, Yamamoto M et al (2008) Proposal for a new clinical entity, IgG4-positive multi-organ lymphoproliferative syndrome: analysis of 64 cases of IgG4-related disorders. Ann Rheum Dis 68:1310–1315. doi:10.1136/ard.2008.089169 (ard.2008.089169 [pii])

Medzhitov R, Janeway C Jr (2000) Innate immunity. N Engl J Med 343(5):338–344. doi:10.1056/NEJM200008033430506

Mukai M, Shinata R, Sugisaki T (2004) Circulating IgG4 anti-IgG4 antibodies in patients with idiopathic membranous nephropathy. Showa Univ J Med Sci 16:289–299

Muraki T, Hamano H, Ochi Y, Komatsu K, Komiyama Y, Arakura N et al (2006) Autoimmune pancreatitis and complement activation system. Pancreas. 32(1):16–21. doi:00006676-200601000-00003 [pii]

Plomp JJ, Huijbers MG, van der Maarel SM, Verschuuren JJ (2012) Pathogenic IgG4 subclass autoantibodies in MuSK myasthenia gravis. Ann NY Acad Sci 1275:114–122. doi:10.1111/j.1749-6632.2012.06808.x

Rispens T, Ooievaar-De Heer P, Vermeulen E, Schuurman J, van der Neut Kolfschoten M, Aalberse RC (2009) Human IgG4 binds to IgG4 and conformationally altered IgG1 via Fc-Fc interactions. J Immunol. 182(7):4275–4281. doi:10.4049/jimmunol.0804338 (182/7/4275 [pii])

Rispens T, Ooijevaar-de Heer P, Bende O, Aalberse RC (2011) Mechanism of immunoglobulin G4 Fab-arm exchange. J Am Chem Soc. 133(26):10302–10311. doi:10.1021/ja203638y

Rock B, Martins CR, Theofilopoulos AN, Balderas RS, Anhalt GJ, Labib RS et al (1989) The pathogenic effect of IgG4 autoantibodies in endemic pemphigus foliaceus (fogo selvagem). N Engl J Med 320(22):1463–1469

Saeki T, Ito T, Yamazaki H, Imai N, Nishi S (2009) Hypocomplementemia of unknown etiology: an opportunity to find cases of IgG4-positive multi-organ lymphoproliferative syndrome. Rheumatol Int. doi:10.1007/s00296-009-0925-4

Saeki T, Nishi S, Imai N, Ito T, Yamazaki H, Kawano M et al (2010) Clinicopathological characteristics of patients with IgG4-related tubulointerstitial nephritis. Kidney Int 78 (10):1016–1023. doi:10.1038/ki.2010.271 (ki2010271 [pii])

Shiokawa M, Kodama Y, Kuriyama K, Yoshimura K, Tomono T, Morita T et al (2016) Pathogenicity of IgG in patients with IgG4-related disease. Gut. doi:10.1136/gutjnl-2015-310336

Shirakata Y, Shiraishi S, Sayama K, Miki Y (1990) Subclass characteristics of IgG autoantibodies in bullous pemphigoid and pemphigus. J Dermatol 17(11):661–666

Stone JH, Zen Y, Deshpande V (2012) IgG4-related disease. N Engl J Med 366(6):539–551. doi:10.1056/NEJMra1104650

Sugimoto M, Watanabe H, Asano T, Sato S, Takagi T, Kobayashi H et al (2016) Possible participation of IgG4 in the activation of complement in IgG4-related disease with hypocomplementemia. Mod Rheumatol 26(2):251–258. doi:10.3109/14397595.2015.1076924

Umehara H, Okazaki K, Masaki Y, Kawano M, Yamamoto M, Saeki T et al (2011) A novel clinical entity, IgG4-related disease (IgG4RD): general concept and details. Mod Rheumatol. doi:10.1007/s10165-011-0508-6

van der Neut Kolfschoten M, Schuurman J, Losen M, Bleeker WK, Martinez-Martinez P, Vermeulen E et al (2007) Anti-inflammatory activity of human IgG4 antibodies by dynamic Fab arm exchange. Science 317(5844):1554–1557. doi:10.1126/science.1144603 (317/5844/1554 [pii])

van der Zee JS, van Swieten P, Aalberse RC (1986) Serologic aspects of IgG4 antibodies. II. IgG4 antibodies form small, nonprecipitating immune complexes due to functional monovalency. J Immunol. 137(11):3566–3571

Wucherpfennig KW, Yu B, Bhol K, Monos DS, Argyris E, Karr RW et al (1995) Structural basis for major histocompatibility complex (MHC)-linked susceptibility to autoimmunity: charged residues of a single MHC binding pocket confer selective presentation of self-peptides in pemphigus vulgaris. Proc Natl Acad Sci USA. 92(25):11935–11939

Yamamoto M, Takahashi H, Ohara M, Suzuki C, Naishiro Y, Yamamoto H et al (2006) A new conceptualization for Mikulicz's disease as an IgG4-related plasmacytic disease. Mod Rheumatol 16(6):335–340. doi:10.1007/s10165-006-0518-Y

Yang Y, Wang C, Jin L, He F, Li C, Gao Q et al (2016) IgG4 anti-phospholipase A2 receptor might activate lectin and alternative complement pathway meanwhile in idiopathic membranous nephropathy: an inspiration from a cross-sectional study. Immunol Res. doi:10.1007/s12026-016-8790-1

Th1/Th2 Immune Balance and Other T Helper Subsets in IgG4-Related Disease

Masafumi Moriyama and Seiji Nakamura

Abstract IgG4-related disease (IgG4-RD) is a systemic disease characterized by elevated serum IgG4 levels and a strong infiltration of IgG4-positive plasma cells in various organs. IgG4-RD patients also frequently suffer from allergic diseases, including asthma and atopic dermatitis. It is well known that T helper type 2 (Th2) cells have an important role in the initiation of allergic diseases, and Th2 cytokines such as interleukin (IL)-4 and IL-13 promote class switching to IgG4. Therefore, IgG4-RD is considered to be a Th2-predominant disease. However, other Th subsets, including regulatory T cells and T follicular helper cells, have recently received increasing attention with regard to the pathogenesis of IgG4-RD. Exploring the interconnected network of Th subsets in IgG4-RD is a highly promising field of investigation. In this review, we focus on the localization and functions of individual Th subsets to clarify the involvement of these cells in the pathogenesis of IgG4-RD.

Contents

Competing interests: The authors declare no competing interests.

M. Moriyama
OCT Research Center, Faculty of Dental Science, Kyushu University, Fukuoka, Japan

S. Nakamura (✉)
Division of Maxillofacial Diagnostic and Surgical Sciences, Section of Oral and Maxillofacial Oncology, Faculty of Dental Science, Kyushu University, 3-1-1 Maidashi, Higashi-ku, Fukuoka 812-8582, Japan
e-mail: seiji@dent.kyushu-u.ac.jp

Current Topics in Microbiology and Immunology (2017) 401: 75–84
DOI 10.1007/82_2016_40

Published Online: 24 September 2016

1 Introduction

IgG4-related disease (IgG4-RD) is a novel clinical entity characterized by severe fibrosis and marked infiltration of IgG4-positive plasma cells with hyperplastic ectopic germinal centers (GCs) in multiple target organs, including the pancreas (Hamano et al. 2001), bile duct (Zen et al. 2004), kidney (Takeda et al. 2004), lung (Zen et al. 2009), lymph nodes (Sato et al. 2009), thyroid (Dahlgren et al. 2010), retroperitoneum (Hamano et al. 2002), and lacrimal and salivary glands (Yamamoto et al. 2005). IgG4-RD has a wide range of presentations, such as autoimmune pancreatitis (AIP), cholangitis, interstitial nephritis, interstitial pneumonitis, lymphadenopathy, Riedel thyroiditis, retroperitoneal fibrosis, and Mikulicz's disease.

Notably, IgG4 is a T helper type 2 (Th2)-dependent immunoglobulin and has low affinity for its target antigen. Th2 cytokines such as interleukin (IL)-4 and IL-10 direct naïve human B cell immunoglobulin isotype switching to IgG4 and IgE production (Meiler et al. 2008). As shown in Fig. 1, at least six subsets of $CD4^+$ Th cells have been identified to date: Th0, Th1, Th2, Th17, regulatory T (Treg), and follicular helper T (Tfh) cells, which are generally considered to maintain homeostasis of the immune system. Interestingly, various diseases may be induced by the impaired regulation of these cells (King et al. 2008). Recent studies suggested that

Fig. 1 $CD4^+$ T helper subsets lineage. *Abbreviations* Th, T helper; Treg, regulatory T; Tfh, follicular helper T; CTL, cytotoxic T cell

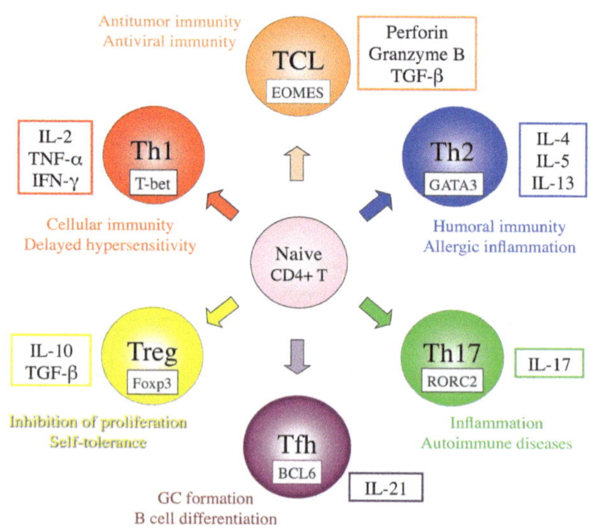

particular Th subsets might be involved in the initiation of IgG4-RD (van der Neut et al. 2007; Rispens et al. 2009). This review will summarize the results of recent studies seeking to understand the role of Th cell subsets in IgG4-RD.

2 Th1/Th2 Balance

Th1 cells produce IL-2, interferon (IFN)-γ, and tumor necrosis factor (TNF)-α, which induce the inflammatory responses responsible for cellular immunity. In contrast, Th2 cells produce IL-4, IL-5, and IL-13, which provide help for humoral immunity. Th2 responses can also counteract Th1-mediated microbicidal action. Many allergic and autoimmune disorders are associated with polarization of the Th1/Th2 balance (Kennedy et al. 1992; Rapoport et al. 1993). IL-4 causes immunoglobulin isotype switching to IgG4 and IgE production (Punnonen et al. 1993). IgG4-RD patients also frequently develop allergic disease, including bronchial asthma, allergic rhinitis, and atopic dermatitis, with severe eosinophilia and elevation of serum IgE levels (Zen et al. 2007). Thus, many studies of this disease suggest that Th2 polarization contributes to the pathogenesis of IgG4-RD (Zen et al. 2007; Tanaka et al. 2012; Nakashima et al. 2010; Maehara et al. 2012b; Miyake et al. 2008). We also previously reported that peripheral $CD4^{+}$ Th cells from patients with IgG4-related dacryoadenitis and sialadenitis (IgG4-DS), so-called Mikulicz's disease, revealed deviation of the Th1/Th2 balance toward Th2 (Miyake et al. 2008). Furthermore, the expression profile of cytokines in salivary glands from patients with IgG4-DS suggested that Th2 immune reactions might play a key role in IgG4 production (Tanaka et al. 2012).

However, the mechanism of Th2 immune activation in IgG4-RD remains to be clarified. In a recent study, we focused on IL-33 as a recently identified cytokine that directly stimulates ST2, the IL-33 receptor, expressed by Th2 cells, eosinophils, and mast cells, to induce production of IL-4, IL-5, and IL-13 (Schmitz et al. 2005). IL-33 is mainly expressed by epithelial cells but also by a wide variety of cell types, including dendritic cells, macrophages, fibroblasts, mast cells, and osteoblasts. Our current data demonstrate that the expression of IL-33 in salivary glands from IgG4-DS patients is significantly higher than that in patients with chronic sialadenitis and healthy controls. Interestingly, the expression of IL-33 in salivary glands was detected around ectopic GCs only in IgG4-DS patients. To confirm the identity of IL-33-producing cells around ectopic GCs, we analyzed the coexpression of immune cell markers and IL-33. The localization of IL-33 was consistent with that of CD163-positive M2 macrophages. In addition, mRNA expression of IL-33 was positively correlated with that of Th2 cytokines only in IgG4-DS patients (manuscript in preparation). These results suggest that the main IL-33 producing cells in IgG4-DS might be M2 macrophages and that they are deeply involved in activation of Th2 immune responses.

In contrast, Okazaki et al. (2000) examined the Th1/Th2 balance in peripheral blood mononuclear cells (PBMCs) in patients with AIP. The number of $CD4^{+}$ Th cells producing IFN-γ and the amount of IFN-γ secreted per cell were significantly increased compared with controls. However, IL-4 was not increased, suggesting that AIP might be mediated by a Th1-predominant immune reaction. With regard to the other organs, several studies reported that IgG4-DS showed a predominance of Th1 cells similar to IgG4-related sclerosing sialadenitis (Ohta et al. 2012). Moreover, Mattoo et al. (2014) analyzed circulating Th2 memory cells and reported that only IgG4-RD patients who had a history of atopic dermatitis showed an increase in circulating Th2 memory cells. They concluded that IgG4-RD promotes Th2 responses resulting from concomitant atopic manifestations. This discrepancy between studies might be explained by the aberrant activation of Th2 responses caused by differences in the severity of the disease or the presence of allergic disease.

3 Other $CD4^+$ T Helper Subsets

3.1 Th17 Cells

The Th1/Th2 paradigm was expanded by the identification of Th17 cells, a subset of $CD4^+$ Th cells characterized by their ability to produce IL-17 and expression of the transcription factor RORγt, and which play a crucial role in the induction of autoimmunity and allergic inflammation by mediating the recruitment of neutrophils and macrophages to affected tissues (Infante-Duarte et al. 2000). Our previous data demonstrated that both Th1 and Th17 cells that infiltrated around ductal epithelial cells might be deeply involved in the initiation of Sjögren's syndrome, a chronic autoimmune disease targeting the exocrine glands, specifically the salivary and lacrimal glands (Moriyama et al. 2012; Maehara et al. 2012b). In contrast, IgG4-DS showed non-periductal lymphocytic infiltration and mild destruction of epithelial cells. However, Th-17-related molecules were rarely seen in the salivary glands (Tanaka et al. 2012; Maehara et al. 2012a). From these findings, we speculate that IgG4-DS might not be a Th17-mediated autoimmune disease.

3.2 Treg Cells

Treg cells are essential for the maintenance of immunological self-tolerance and immune homeostasis by direct contact with effector immune cells or by the secretion of anti-inflammatory cytokines, such as IL-10 and transforming growth factor (TGF)-β. Treg cells exert their effects through the modulation of both T and B cell responses, and two subsets of Treg cells, $CD4^+$ $CD25^+$ $Foxp3^+$ Treg cells and

IL-10-producing Tr1 cells, play a key role in regulating effector T cell functions (Shevach et al. 2006).

Allergic immune responses develop in response to the Th2 cytokines IL-4 and IL-13, which are responsible for IgG4 and IgE production by B cells. Interestingly, it was shown that the class switching to IgG4 is caused by co-stimulation with IL-4 and IL-10 and that IL-10 decreased the switching of IL-4-induced IgE but elevated the switching of IL-4-induced IgG4. This specific isotype switching is regarded as a 'modified Th2 response' (Maizels and Yazdanbakhsh 2003). Zen et al. (2007) reported that $CD4^+$ $CD25^+$ $Foxp3^+$ Treg cells strongly infiltrated into the affected tissues and produced IL-10 and TGF-β in cases of IgG4-related sclerosing pancreatitis and cholangitis. In addition, we found that mRNA expression of IL-4, IL-10, and Foxp3 in salivary glands from patients with IgG4-DS was positively correlated with the IgG4/IgG ratio obtained immunohistochemically (Tanaka et al. 2012). These results suggest that Th2 and regulatory immune reactions might promote B cells to produce IgG4.

3.3 Tfh Cells

Tfh cells were identified as a unique Th phenotype, contributing to isotype switching, somatic hypermutation, and GC formation. Several studies reported that Tfh cells control the functional activity of effector Th cells and promote ectopic GC formation via IL-21, which impairs B cell differentiation (Vinuesa et al. 2010). IL-4 and IL-21 receptor knockout mice have significantly reduced IgG responses, indicating that IL-21 cooperates with IL-4 to regulate humoral immune responses (Ozaki et al. 2002). Furthermore, IL-21 directly inhibits IL-4-induced IgE production and induces the switching to IgG4 by co-stimulation with IL-4 and IL-21 (Kitayama et al. 2008). We previously found that expression of IL-21 correlated with the number of GCs formed in salivary glands from patients with IgG4-DS, further suggesting that aberrant IL-21 production might induce multiple GC formation and the switching of IgG4.

Recent studies demonstrated that the Tfh population comprises functionally distinct subsets characterized by specific patterns of surface antigens and that at least three subsets exist: Tfh1, Tfh2, and Tfh17 cells (Morita et al. 2011). Tfh1 cells secrete IFN-γ upon activation and have limited class switching activity. Tfh2 and Tfh17 cells induce the switching of various immunoglobulin isotypes (IgM, IgA, IgG, and IgE). Akiyama et al. (2015) reported that the number of circulating Tfh2 cells was increased in IgG4-RD and correlated with the number of plasmablasts and serum IgG4 and IL-4 levels. Moreover, the number of plasmablasts and levels of serum IgG4 and IL-4 decreased after glucocorticoid treatment, while that of Tfh2 cells remained unchanged. They concluded that Tfh2 cells are the underlying pathogenic T cell population in IgG4-RD.

3.4 CD4⁺ CTL Cells

Cytotoxic $CD4^+$ T cells ($CD4^+$ CTLs) are characterized by the production of IFN-γ, granzyme B, and perforin, and are distinct from any conventional $CD4^+$ Th subset (Van de Berg et al. 2008). Mattoo et al. (2016) reported that circulating $CD4^+$ CTLs were clonally expanded in IgG4-RD and the dominant T cells in disease tissues. The circulating $CD4^+$ $SLAMF7^+$ CTLs in IgG4-RD patients declines concomitant with a clinical response to rituximab therapy. In addition, the ratio of $CD4^+$ $GraB^+$ CTLs in IgG4-DS lesions was positively correlated with the serum IgG4 levels, as well as the number of affected organs. This suggests that the dysregulation of $CD4^+$ CTLs might play a key role in the pathogenesis of IgG4-RD.

4 Conclusions

The physiological role of IgG4 antibody in IgG4-RD is poorly understood. IgG4 antibodies are generally considered to have a poor ability to activate complement and immune complex formation, which leads to anti-inflammatory activity. Moreover, specific antigens recognized by IgG4 have yet to be identified. From these findings, we speculate that the aberrant IgG4 production in IgG4-RD does not behave as a tissue-destructive immunoglobulin, but as a secondary reactive response induced by a unique cytokine milieu (Fig. 2).

Innate immunity has recently received much attention regarding the initiation of IgG4-RD. Several studies indicated that abnormal innate immune responses via toll-like receptors (TLRs) expressed by monocytes/macrophage enhanced Th2 immune responses and the immunopathogenesis of IgG4-RDs (Watanabe et al. 2012; Fukui et al. 2015). Macrophages are known to play an important role in the immune response to foreign substances or microbes by presenting pathogen antigens to antigen-specific Th cells. Notably, M2 macrophages scavenge debris and contribute to angiogenesis, wound healing, and fibrosis by producing IL-10 and CCL18 (Van Gorp et al. 2010). Thus, we have analyzed the relationships between M2 macrophages and the initiation of IgG4-RD and demonstrated the predominant infiltration of M2 macrophages in affected lesions from patients with IgG4-RD (Furukawa et al. 2015). In our latest study, we performed microarray analysis of gene expression in salivary gland samples to identify innate immune molecules and found that macrophage receptor with collagenous structure (MARCO) was identified as a disease-associated molecule in IgG4-RD. Moreover, the expression pattern of MARCO was consistent with that of the M2 macrophage marker CD163 (Ohta et al. 2016).

Thus, research accumulated in recent years has enhanced our understanding of the immunological background of IgG4-RD. However, additional research is still required to further elucidate the pathogenesis of IgG4-DS, especially the connection between innate and adaptive immunity.

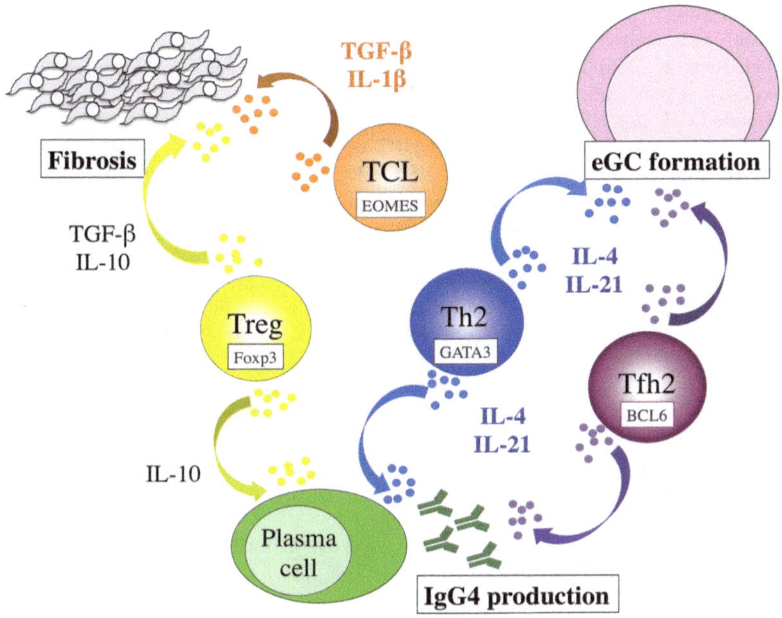

Fig. 2 Schematic model of Th subsets in IgG4-RD. Th2, Treg, and Tfh2 cells play key roles in GC formation and IgG4 production. Treg cells and $CD4^+$ CTLs promote local fibrosis by IL-1β and TGF-β

Funding This work was supported in part by grants from the Ministry of Education, Culture, Sports, Science, and Technology of Japan (26293430, 26670869), the 'Research on Measures for Intractable Diseases' project, a matching fund subsidy from the Ministry of Health Labour and Welfare, Japan (H26-026, H26-064), the 'Practical Research Project for Rare/Intractable Diseases,' a matching fund subsidy from the Japan Agency for Medical Research and Development (H26-275, H26-313).

References

Akiyama M, Suzuki K, Yamaoka K et al (2015) Number of circulating follicular helper 2 T Cells correlates with IgG4 and Interleukin-4 levels and plasmablast numbers in IgG4-related disease. Arthritis Rheumatol 67(9):2476–2481

Dahlgren M, Khosroshahi A, Nielsen GP et al (2010) Riedel's thyroiditis and multifocal fibrosclerosis are part of the IgG4-related systemic disease spectrum. Arthritis Care Res 62 (9):1312–1318

Fukui Y, Uchida K, Sakaguchi Y et al (2015) Possible involvement of Toll-like receptor 7 in the development of type 1 autoimmune pancreatitis. J Gastroenterol 50(4):435–444

Furukawa S, Moriyama M, Tanaka A et al (2015) Preferential M2 macrophages contribute to fibrosis in IgG4-related dacryoadenitis and sialoadenitis, so-called Mikulicz's disease. Clin Immunol 156(1):9–18

Hamano H, Kawa S, Horiuchi A et al (2001) High serum IgG4 concentrations in patients with sclerosing pancreatitis. N Engl J Med 344(10):732–738

Hamano H, Kawa S, Ochi Y et al (2002) Hydronephrosis associated with retroperitoneal fibrosis and sclerosing pancreatitis. Lancet 359(9315):1403–1404

Infante-Duarte C, Horton HF, Byrne MC et al (2000) Microbial lipopeptides induce the production of IL-17 in Th cells. J Immunol 165(11):6107–6115

Kennedy MK, Torrance DS, Picha KS et al (1992) Analysis of cytokine mRNA expression in the central nervous system of mice with experimental autoimmune encephalomyelitis reveals that IL-10 mRNA expression correlates with recovery. J Immunol 149(7):2496–2505

King C, Tangye SG, Mackay CR (2008) T follicular helper (TFH) cells in normal and dysregulated immune responses. Annu Rev Immunol 26:741–766

Kitayama D, Sakamoto A, Arima M et al (2008) A role for Bcl6 in sequential class switch recombination to IgE in B cells stimulated with IL-4 and IL-21. Mol Immunol 45(5): 1337–1345

Maehara T, Moriyama M, Nakashima H et al (2012a) Interleukin-21 contributes to germinal centre formation and immunoglobulin G4 production in IgG4-related dacryoadenitis and sialoadenitis, so-called Mikulicz's disease. Ann Rheum Dis 71(12):2011–2020

Maehara T, Moriyama M, Hayashida JN et al (2012b) Selective localization of T helper subsets in labial salivary glands from primary Sjogren's syndrome patients. Clin Exp Immunol 169: 89–99

Maizels RM, Yazdanbakhsh M (2003) Immune regulation by helminth parasites: cellular and molecular mechanisms. Nat Rev Immunol 3(9):733–744

Mattoo H, Mahajan VS, Della-Torre E et al (2014) De novo oligoclonal expansions of circulating plasmablasts in active and relapsing IgG4-related disease. J Allergy Clin Immunol 134(3): 679–687

Mattoo H, Mahajan VS, Maehara T et al (2016) Clonal expansion of $CD4^+$ cytotoxic T lymphocytes in IgG4-related disease. J Allergy Clin Immunol

Meiler F, Klunker S, Zimmermann M et al (2008) Distinct regulation of IgE, IgG4 and IgA by T regulatory cells and toll-like receptors. Allergy 63(11):1455–1463

Miyake K, Moriyama M, Aizawa K et al (2008) Peripheral $CD4^+$ T cells showing a Th2 phenotype in a patient with Mikulicz's disease associated with lymphadenopathy and pleural effusion. Mod Rheumatol 18(1):86–90

Morita R, Schmitt N, Bentebibel SE et al (2011) Human blood CXCR5(+)CD4(+) T cells are counterparts of T follicular cells and contain specific subsets that differentially support antibody secretion. Immunity 34(1):108–121

Moriyama M, Hayashida JN, Toyoshima T et al (2012) Cytokine/chemokine profiles contribute to understanding the pathogenesis and diagnosis of primary Sjogren's syndrome. Clin Exp Immunol 169:17–26

Nakashima H, Miyake K, Moriyama M et al (2010) An amplification of IL-10 and TGF-beta in patients with IgG4-related tubulointerstitial nephritis. Clin Nephrol 73(5):385–391

Ohta N, Makihara S, Okano M et al (2012) Roles of IL-17, Th1, and Tc1 cells in patients with IgG4-related sclerosing sialadenitis. Laryngoscope 122(10):2169–2174

Ohta M, Moriyama M, Maehara T et al (2016) DNA microarray analysis of submandibular glands in IgG4-related disease indicates a role for MARCO and other innate immune related proteins. Medicine 95(7):e2853

Okazaki K, Uchida K, Ohana M et al (2000) Autoimmune-related pancreatitis is associated with autoantibodies and a Thl/Th2-type cellular immune response. Gastroenterology 118(3): 573–581

Ozaki K, Spolski R, Feng CG et al (2002) A critical role for IL-21 in regulating immunoglobulin production. Science 298(5598):1630–1634

Punnonen J, Aversa G, Cocks BG et al (1993) Interleukin 13 induces interleukin 4-independent IgG4 and IgE synthesis and CD23 expression by human B cells. Proc Natl Acad Sci USA 90 (8):3730–3734

Rapoport MJ, Jaramillo A, Zipris D et al (1993) Interleukin 4 reverses T cell proliferative unresponsiveness and prevents the onset of diabetes in nonobese diabetic mice. J Exp Med 178 (1):87–99

Rispens T, Ooievaar-De Heer P, Vermeulen E et al (2009) Human IgG4 binds to IgG4 and conformationally altered IgG1 via Fc-Fc interactions. J Immunol 182(7):4275–4281

Sato Y, Kojima M, Takata K et al (2009) Systemic IgG4-related lymphadenopathy: a clinical and pathologic comparison to multicentric Castleman's disease. Mod Pathol 22(4):589–599

Schmitz J, Owyang A, Oldham E et al (2005) IL-33, an interleukin-1-like cytokine that signals via the IL-1 receptor-related protein ST2 and induces T helper type 2-associated cytokines. Immunity 23:479–490

Shevach EM, DiPaolo RA, Andersson J et al (2006) The lifestyle of naturally occurring $CD4^+$ $CD25^+$ $Foxp3^+$ regulatory T cells. Immunol Rev 212:60–73

Takeda S, Haratake J, Kasai T et al (2004) IgG4-associated idiopathic tubulointerstitial nephritis complicating autoimmune pancreatitis. Nephrol Dial Transplant 19(2):474–476

Tanaka A, Moriyama M, Nakashima H et al (2012) Th2 and regulatory immune reactions contribute to IgG4 production and the initiation of Mikulicz disease. Arthritis Rheum 64 (1):254–263

Van de Berg PJ, van Leeuwen E, ten Berge IJ et al (2008) Cytotoxic human $CD4^+$ T cells. Curr Opin Immunol 20:339–343

van der Neut Kolfschoten M, Schuurman J, Losen M et al (2007) Anti-inflammatory activity of human IgG4 antibodies by dynamic Fab arm exchange. Science 317(5844):1554–1557

Van Gorp H, Delputte PL, Nauwynck HJ (2010) Scavenger receptor CD163, a Jack-of-all-trades and potential target for cell-directed therapy. Mol Immunol 47:1650–1660

Vinuesa CG, Linterman MA, Goodnow CC et al (2010) T cells and follicular dendritic cells in germinal center B-cell formation and selection. Immunol Rev 237(1):72–89

Watanabe T, Yamashita K, Fujikawa S et al (2012) Involvement of activation of toll-like receptors and nucleotide-binding oligomerization domain-like receptors in enhanced IgG4 responses in autoimmune pancreatitis. Arthritis Rheumatol 64(3):914–924

Yamamoto M, Harada S, Ohara M et al (2005) Clinical and pathological differences between Mikulicz's disease and Sjogren's syndrome. Rheumatology 44(2):227–234

Zen Y, Harada K, Sasaki M et al (2004) IgG4-related sclerosing cholangitis with and without hepatic inflammatory pseudotumor, and sclerosing pancreatitis-associated sclerosing cholangitis: do they belong to a spectrum of sclerosing pancreatitis? Am J Surg Pathol 28(9): 1193–1203

Zen Y, Fujii T, Harada K et al (2007) Th2 and regulatory immune reactions are increased in immunoglobin G4-related sclerosing pancreatitis and cholangitis. Hepatology 45(6): 1538–1546

Zen Y, Inoue D, Kitao A et al (2009) IgG4-related lung and pleural disease: a clinicopathologic study of 21 cases. Am J Surg Pathol 33(12):1886–1893

Roles of Plasmablasts and B Cells in IgG4-Related Disease: Implications for Therapy and Early Treatment Outcomes

Marco Lanzillotta, Emanuel Della-Torre and John H. Stone

Abstract High serum IgG4 concentrations are a striking feature of many patients with IgG4-related disease (IgG4-RD). Blood levels of IgG4 often reach ten, twenty, and even thirty or more times higher than the upper limit of normal. Under the proper clinical circumstances, the finding of an elevated serum IgG4 concentration serves as a useful biomarker for the diagnosis of this condition. This serum IgG4 elevation quickly called attention to the possibility of therapies targeting cells of the B lymphocyte lineage. In addition, a greater understanding of the cellular mechanisms that underpin IgG4-RD has identified peripheral blood plasmablasts as a promising biomarker for this disease. The roles of plasmablasts and B cells in IgG4-RD are discussed in this chapter.

Contents

M. Lanzillotta · E. Della-Torre
Unit of Medicine and Clinical Immunology, IRCCS San Raffaele Scientific Institute, Università Vita-Salute San Raffaele, Milan, Italy

J.H. Stone (✉)
Harvard Medical School, Clinical Rheumatology, Massachusetts General Hospital, Boston, MA, USA
e-mail: jhstone@mgh.harvard.edu

Current Topics in Microbiology and Immunology (2017) 401: 85–92
DOI 10.1007/82_2016_58

Published Online: 05 January 2017

1 Introduction

The high serum IgG4 concentrations in many patients with IgG4-related disease (IgG4-RD)—sometimes reaching levels several dozen times the upper limit of normal—have suggested an important role for humoral immunity since the earliest days of this condition's recognition (Hamano et al. 2001). The range of IgG4 concentrations in IgG4-RD is broad, however: some patients have serum IgG4 concentrations thirty to forty times the upper limit of normal, yet up to 40% of patients with biopsy-proven disease have normal serum IgG4 concentrations (Wallace et al. 2016). The fact that only an imperfect relationship exists between serum IgG4 concentrations and changes in disease activity suggests more at play than humoral immunity alone, but both the clinical results of treatment trials and findings from mechanistic studies indicate a crucial contribution from cells of the B-cell lineage in IgG4-RD. In this chapter, the roles of B cells and plasmablasts—critical players in disease pathophysiology and leading targets for therapy—are considered.

2 A Short Summary of B-Cell Development

The B lymphocyte lineage encompasses a broad spectrum of cell subsets that differ in their morphology, surface markers, and biologic function. CD20, a unique B-cell antigen, is first expressed on cells of the B-lymphocyte lineage in the bone marrow, at the pre-B stage, and continues to be expressed through the memory B-cell stage. The CD20 antigen is lost at some imprecisely defined point during the maturation of fully developed B cells into plasma cells, through the intermediary stage of plasmablasts. Understanding of the functions of CD20 remains incomplete, but this antigen is believed to play a role in B-cell receptor-mediated signaling (Fink 2012). Rituximab, a chimeric monoclonal antibody, targets CD20, leading to the depletion of all components of the B-lymphocyte lineage beginning with the pre-B stage and extending through the stage of mature B cells.

CD19, also known as the B-lymphocyte antigen, is present on an even broader spectrum of the B-cell lineage than is CD20. CD19, found on the earliest recognizable B-lineage cells up to and including plasmablast stage, is no longer present on mature plasma cells. The primary function of CD19 is as a co-receptor in conjunction with CD21 and CD81 for the recruitment of phosphatidyl inositol kinases following cellular activation (Fink 2012). During their maturation process from $CD19^{+}$ naïve B cells into plasmablasts, cells of the B-cell lineage alter their phenotype through the down-regulation of certain surface markers—particularly CD20—and the up-regulation of others, e.g., CD27 and CD38. Plasmablasts, which appear as $CD19^{low}CD20^{-}CD27^{+}CD38^{bright}$ cells within a population of $CD45^{bright}$side-$scatter^{low}$ leucocytes, are identifiable by flow cytometry and constitute a useful marker of disease activity.

Plasmablasts, positioned between activated naïve/memory B cells and antibody-secreting plasma cells in the cellular maturation of the B lineage, represent a transitional stage of the B cell. Naïve B-lymphocytes differentiate from hematopoietic stem cells in the bone marrow, where they undergo their initial V-D-J and V-J rearrangements in the creation of immunoglobulin heavy and light chains genes, respectively. This process results in the expression of a fully functional B-cell receptor, enabling naïve B cells to recognize specific protein antigens. Naïve B cells exit the bone marrow and migrate to secondary lymphoid organs, e.g., the lymph nodes and spleen, the sites at which antigen recognition occurs.

Antigen recognition through the B-cell receptor activates naïve B cells. A cascade of immunological events is triggered thereby, culminating in antigen-specific expansions not only of B cells but also of T cell populations. Activated, antigen-primed naïve B-cells undergo a process known as somatic mutation, which consists of further rounds of V-D-J segments rearrangements. Somatic hypermutation heightens both the affinity and the specificity of antibodies secreted by these cells. In addition to their eventual roles in humoral immunity as antibody-producing cells following their transition to plasma cells, however, activated B-cells also play critical roles as antigen-presenting cells for naïve T cells, thus facilitating cell-mediated immune responses.

Following somatic mutation, activated B-cells migrate within the germinal centers, where they re-encounter their cognate antigen presented by resident follicular dendritic cells. B cells that fail to recognize the antigen die. Those B cells with the highest antigen affinities, however, survive and proliferate as they move toward the next step of development, affinity maturation, which consists of additional mutations and antigen-mediated affinity checking (Kepler and Perelson 1993). This process ensures the production of antibodies with high antigen specificity (Allen et al. 2007). Class switch recombination, a process in which activated B-cells switch the heavy chain isotypes of their antibodies (IgG, IgE, or IgA) under the guidance of contact or soluble signals from helper T cells, also occurs within germinal centers (McHeyzer-Williams and McHeyzer-Williams 2005).

Memory B cells and plasmablasts take divergent paths after completing somatic mutation, affinity maturation, and class-switching. Memory B cells exit the secondary lymphoid organs and re-circulate in the peripheral blood. They migrate back to other antigen-draining tissues (e.g., other lymph node chains), where they retain the capability of rapidly differentiating into plasmablasts in anticipation of be called upon to do so in the context of re-exposure to their cognate antigens.

In contrast, plasmablasts, which are not distinguishable morphologically on blood smear from small-sized, activated lymphocytes, circulate briefly in the peripheral blood on their way back to either the bone marrow or tissue inflammation, where they complete their differentiation into plasma cells (Hiepe et al. 2011). Although plasmablasts express many chemokine receptors that enable their attraction by soluble molecules within specific niches (Chavele et al. 2015), the vast majority of plasmablasts die within days—the result of failure to identify appropriate survival niches.

Healthy individuals have only low levels of plasmablasts detectable in the peripheral blood—potentially observed following vaccination or an active infection. In the setting of chronic immune-mediated condition, however, e.g., IgG4-RD, systemic lupus erythematosus, inflammatory bowel disease, or rheumatoid arthritis, plasmablasts can circulate for prolonged periods and achieve high blood concentrations. Resident plasma cells, in contrast, express adhesion molecules (e.g., CD138) and lose the migratory capabilities characteristic of cells in earlier stages of B-cell development (Kaminski et al. 2012).

Plasmablasts retain the capabilities of dividing, of presenting antigens to T cells through MHC class II molecules, and of interacting with T cells through the B7 and CD40 surface antigens. In fact, plasmablasts have a fundamental role within germinal centers in the induction of T follicular helper cell differentiation. This step, driven by IL-6, is crucial for appropriate B-cell development and affinity maturation (Chavele et al. 2015).

3 Plasmablasts in IgG4-Related Disease

Next-generation sequencing studies on B cells from the peripheral blood of IgG4-RD patients have led to the identification of an expanded population of circulating, antigen-specific plasmablasts (Mattoo et al. 2014). Similarly, the oligoclonally expanded $IgG4^{+}$ cells that surround lymphoid follicles in the secondary or tertiary lymphoid organs of patients with IgG4-RD are $CD19^{+}CD20^{-}$, and therefore represent either tissue plasmablasts or plasma cells.

The concentrations of plasmablasts, which appear as $CD19^{low}CD20^{-}CD27^{+}$ $CD38^{bright}$ cells on flow cytometry, are present in numbers dramatically higher in IgG4-RD patients compared to those observed in health individuals (Mattoo et al. 2014). Plasmablasts in IgG4-RD also show low levels of surface IgM but high levels of IgG4, HLA-DR, BCMA, and SLAMF7, a CD2 family receptor expressed on activated human B cells. Mattoo and colleagues demonstrated that the expanded plasmablast pool in IgG4-RD patients decreases sharply following anti-CD20 treatment (Mattoo et al. 2014), corresponding to the induction of clinical remission. These plasmablasts re-emerge during relapse and their concentrations correlate more closely with disease activity than do serum IgG4 levels (Wallace et al. 2014).

Increased levels of $CD19^{low}CD20^{-}CD27^{+}CD38^{bright}$ cells are reported in IgG4-RD patients with active disease whose serum IgG4 concentrations are normal—but the converse does not appear to be true. Thus, a low blood plasmablast concentration supports a state of disease quiescence. If observed before treatment, a low plasmablast concentrations urge the search for other diagnoses. Wallace et al., in an investigation of the test characteristic of circulating plasmablasts as biomarkers, use a cut-off value for the upper limit of normal for plasmablast concentrations of 900 cells/mL. They reported a sensitivity of 95%, a specificity of 82%, a positive predictive value of 86%, and a negative predictive value of 97% for diagnostic purposes (Wallace et al. 2014). These findings require confirmation in larger numbers of IgG4-RD patients and appropriate controls. The utility of $IgG4^+$ plasmablast concentrations as clinical biomarkers is also worth exploring. The reliable measurement of $IgG4^+$ plasmablasts by flow cytometry, however, has challenges pertaining to the stainability of such cells.

A key point about plasmablasts at the time of disease flare is that the re-emergent plasmablasts express V-J repertoires distinct from those of the plasmablasts present during the earlier, pre-treatment phase, a phenomenon known as "clonal divergence" (Mattoo et al. 2014). The fact of clonal divergence suggests repeated rounds of mutation and selection driven by a specific antigen, thereby strongly supporting the concept of IgG4-RD as an antigen-driven condition.

4 How Do B Cells and Plasmablasts Fit into the Overall Pathophysiologic Scheme?

Recent evidence suggests that T-cells play a central role in IgG4-RD pathogenesis. $CD4^+$ T-cells, the most abundant cell within affected tissues, are dispersed throughout IgG4-RD lesions (Deshpande et al. 2012). A clonally expanded population of $CD4^+$ cytotoxic T lymphocytes in both the peripheral blood and fibrotic lesions of IgG4-RD patients suggest that these cells are central to the disease (Mattoo et al. 2016). These cytotoxic T cells elaborate granzyme B and perforin, products more commonly associated with $CD8^+$ T cells. They also produce interleukin-1, transforming growth factor beta, and interferon-gamma, all of which may contribute substantially to the storiform fibrosis that characterizes IgG4-RD.

Given the phenotype and capabilities of this $CD4^+$ cytotoxic T cell, a logical role for both B cells and plasmablasts in the disease pathophysiology is the sustenance of these $CD4^+$ cytotoxic T cells through the continuous presentation of antigen. A T-follicular helper cell response that is separate from the $CD4^+$ cytotoxic T lymphocytes is likely to be responsible for the development of germinal centers within lymph nodes (and involved organs). The T-follicular helper cells could produce the cytokines (e.g., IL-4) that drive the IgG4 class-switch, culminating in the creation of IgG4-secreting plasmablasts and long-lived plasma cells. A number of specific aspects require experimental confirmation.

5 Lessons from Mechanistic Studies

The rapidity with which the serum IgG4 concentration declines following B-cell depletion suggests that the cells making the preponderance of serum IgG4 are short-lived plasmablasts and plasma cells. Plasmablasts decline swiftly following anti-CD20 treatment. Because plasmablasts do not possess the CD20 antigen, one would predict a lack of response to anti-CD20 treatment. On the contrary, the concentration of plasmablasts falls swiftly following B-cell depletion. The explanation for this finding appears to be not direct killing of plasmablasts, but rather to the short-lived nature of the plasmablasts that contribute to IgG4-RD and depletion of their pool of $CD20^+$ progenitors—either naïve B cells or memory B cells. The short-lived plasmablasts and plasma cells cannot be repleted on schedule following their anticipated demise because their B-cell precursors no longer exist. The fact that B-cell depletion does not lead to the complete normalization of serum IgG4 concentrations implies the presence of long-lived plasma cells that continue to make this immunoglobulin.

Iwata et al. (2012) reported a similar drop in peripheral plasmablast count with the use of glucocorticoid therapy alone. However, the memory B-cell count appeared to be unaffected by this treatment, therefore partly explaining why the maintenance of remission in IgG4-RD often fails during glucocorticoid withdrawal.

6 Therapeutic Efforts Targeting the B-Cell Lineage to Date

6.1 Targeting CD20

The efficacy of anti-CD20 in a number of other immune-mediated conditions, including many associated with autoantibodies, made rituximab a logical therapeutic approach for IgG4-RD, a disease in which humoral immunity was believed to play such an important role in the early years after the first description. Rituximab is known to be effective in diseases such as rheumatoid arthritis, ANCA-associated vasculitis, and pemphigus vulgaris. Among the earliest patients in whom rituximab was employed was a 55 year-old man with IgG4-related Mikulicz' disease whose disease had previously been refractory to both prednisone and methotrexate (Khosroshahi et al. 2010). Striking clinical and serological improvement was observed within weeks in that patient following two 1 g administrations of rituximab, each accompanied by methylprednisolone 100 mg.

In a follow-up study, ten patients with IgG4-RD were treated with two doses of RTX (1000 mg each), administered 15 days apart (Khosroshahi et al. 2012). All ten patients discontinued prednisone and other therapies entirely following rituximab treatment. Nine of the 10 patients demonstrated striking clinical improvement within one month of starting rituximab. Only a patient with IgG4-related Riedel's thyroiditis and advanced thyroid fibrosis failed to respond.

A prospective, open-label trial provided further evidence of the efficacy of B-cell depletion (Carruthers et al. 2015). Twenty-six of the 30 patients in that trial were treated with the combination of rituximab (1 g) and methylprednisolone (100 mg), both administered in two doses spaced over two weeks. Only one patient—a patient who repleted his B-cell population only two months after achieving a transient B-cell depletion—failed to demonstrated a clinical response. Nearly half (47%) of the patients were in complete remission at six months, and 40% were in remission one year after treatment despite receiving no consolidation or remission maintenance therapy.

Rituximab-induced remissions are known to be of variable duration, sometimes lasting two years or longer but occasionally being as short as 3–4 months. High baseline serum concentrations of IgG4 and IgE and high baseline blood levels of eosinophils as risk factors for disease relapse (Wallace et al. 2016).

6.2 Targeting CD19

More recent efforts at targeting the B-cell lineage have focused on downregulation and functional inhibition rather than depletion of B cells. One novel therapy known as XmAb5871 targets CD19, therefore affecting in theory a broader population of the B-cell pool compared with anti-CD20 treatment. XmAb5871 takes advantage of the fact that Fc-gamma-RIIb, a down-regulatory Fc-gamma receptor, is the only Fc-gamma receptor on B cells. The implication of this is that co-ligation of Fc-gamma-RIIb along with another cell surface receptor, e.g., CD19, leads to blockade of signaling through the B-cell receptor and inhibition of the cell's function. XmAb5871, a humanized anti-CD19 antibody, possesses an Fc portion engineered to possess an affinity for Fc-gamma-RIIb 200- to 400-fold greater than that of native IgG.

XmAb5871 is presently being tested in a phase 2 clinical trial, an open-label investigation of XmAb5871 in active IgG4-RD. The investigational agent is administered intravenously at a dose of 5 mg/kg every 14 days for 12 doses. Positron emission tomography (PET) scans are performed at baseline and at three months. Glucocorticoids are permitted but not required at entry and must be discontinued by two months. Other immunosuppressive medications are not allowed. Reporting of results from this trial is anticipated in early 2017.

References

Allen CDC, Okada T, Cyster JG (2007) Germinal-center organization and cellular dynamics. Immunity 27(2):190–202

Carruthers MN, Topazian MD, Khosroshahi A, Witzig TE, Wallace ZS, Hart PA, Deshpande V, Smyrk TC, Chari S, Stone JH (2015) Rituximab for IgG4-related disease: a prospective, open-label trial. Ann Rheum Dis 74:1171–1177

Chavele K-M, Merry E, Ehrenstein MR (2015) Cutting edge: circulating plasmablasts induce the differentiation of human T follicular helper cells via IL-6 production. J Immunol 194(6):2482–2485

Deshpande V, Zen Y, Chan JK, Yi EE, Sato Y, Yoshino T et al (2012) Consensus statement on the pathology of IgG4-related disease. Mod Pathol 25:1181–1192

Engel P, Zhou LJ, Ord DC, Sato S, Koller B, Tedder TF (1995) Abnormal B lymphocyte development, activation, and differentiation in mice that lack or overexpress the CD19 signal transduction molecule. Immunity 3:39–50

Fink K (2012) Origin and function of circulating plasmablasts during acute viral infections. Front Immunol 3:78

Iwata S, Saito K, Hirata S, Tanaka Y (2012) Phenotypic changes of lymphocyte in a patient with IgG4-related disease after corticosteroid therapy. Ann Rheum Dis 71(12):2058–2059

Hamano H, Kawa S, Horiuchi A et al (2001) High serum IgG4 concentrations in patients with sclerosing pancreatitis. N Engl J Med 344:732–738

Hiepe F, Dörner T, Hauser AE, Hoyer BF, Mei H, Radbruch A (2011) Long-lived autoreactive plasma cells drive persistent autoimmune inflammation. Nat Rev Rheumatol 7:170–178

Kaminski DA, Wei C, Qian Y, Rosenberg AF, Sanz I (2012) Advances in human B cell phenotypic profiling. Front Immunol 3:302

Kepler TB, Perelson AS (1993) Cyclic re-entry of germinal center B cells and the efficiency of affinity maturation. Immunol Today 14(8):412–415

Khosroshahi A, Bloch DB, Deshpande V, Stone JH (2010) Rituximab therapy leads to swift decline of serum IgG4 levels and prompt clinical improvement in IgG4-related disease. Arthritis Rheum 62:1755–1762

Khosroshahi A, Carruthers MD, Deshpande V et al (2012) Rituximab for the treatment of IgG4-related systemic disease: lessons from a series of ten consecutive cases. Medicine (Baltimore) 91:57–66

Mattoo H, Mahajan VS, Della-Torre E, Sekigami Y, Carruthers M, Wallace ZS et al (2014) De novo oligoclonal expansions of circulating plasmablasts in active and relapsing IgG4-related disease. J Allergy Clin Immunol 13:679–687

Mattoo H, Mahajan VS, Maehara T, Deshpande V, Della-Torre E, Wallace ZS, Kulikova M, Drijvers JM, Daccache J, Carruthers MN, Castellino F, Stone JR, Stone JH, Pillai S (2016) Clonal expansion of CD4 cytotoxic T lymphocytes in patients with IgG-related disease. J Allergy Clin Immunol 138:825–838

McHeyzer-Williams LJ, McHeyzer-Williams MG (2005) Antigen-specific memory B cell development. Annu Rev Immunol 23:487–513

Wallace ZS, Mattoo H, Carruthers M, Mahajan VS, Della Torre E, Lee H et al (2014) Plasmablasts as a biomarker for IgG4-related disease, independent of serum IgG4 concentrations. Ann Rheum Dis 1–6

Wallace ZS, Mattoo H, Mahajan VS, Kulikova M, Lu L, Deshpande V, Choi HK, Pillai S, Stone JH (2016a) Predictors of disease relapse in IgG4-related disease. Rheumatology 55 (6):1000–1008

Wallace ZS, Mattoo H, Mahajan VS, Kulikova M, Lu L, Deshpande V, Choi HK, Pillai S, Stone JH (2016b) Predictors of disease relapse in IgG4-related disease. Rheumatology 55 (6):1000–1008

Roles of Regulatory T and B Cells in IgG4-Related Disease

Kazushige Uchida and Kazuichi Okazaki

Abstract Immunoglobulin G4 (IgG4)-related disease (RD) is a newly recognized systemic disease. Although there are several forms of IgG4-RD reported under various names, depending on the target organ and characteristics, patients with IgG4-RD manifest several immunologic and histologic abnormalities including increased levels of serum IgG4 and storiform fibrosis with infiltration of lymphocytes and IgG4-positive plasmacytes in the involved organs. However, the pathophysiology remains unclear. Regulatory immune cells play an important role in several immune-related diseases. In particular, abnormalities in regulatory T cell (Treg) and regulatory B cell (Breg) numbers and function are implicated in several immune-related (include autoimmune) conditions, and their roles in IgG4-RD have recently begun to be investigated. We provide an overview of the research conducted to date on Tregs and Bregs in IgG4-RD. We highlight the basic functions of these cells, their changes in patients with various forms of IgG4-RD, and insight gained from animal models of the disease. Based on the evidence accumulated thus far, we proposed a hypothesis for the pathophysiological mechanism of IgG4-RD with respect to the roles regulatory immune cells, and highlight the questions and venues of research deserving of further attenuation, Over all, we demonstrate that Tregs and Bregs have a clear impact on IgG4-RD, and further exploration of this field is expected to lead to a better mechanistic understanding of the disease, hopefully resulting in the in the discovery of new therapeutic targets.

K. Uchida (✉)
Department of Gastroenterology and Hepatology, Kansai Medical University,
2-5-1 Shinmachi, Hirakata 573-1197, Osaka, Japan
e-mail: uchidak@hirakata.kmu.ac.jp

K. Uchida · K. Okazaki
Department of Gastroenterology and Hepatology, Kansai Medical University,
Hirakata, Japan

Current Topics in Microbiology and Immunology (2017) 401: 93–114
DOI 10.1007/82_2016_41

Published Online: 05 November 2016

Contents

1 Introduction

Immunoglobulin G4-related disease (IgG4-RD) is a newly recognized systemic inflammatory condition that is characterized by lymphoplasmacytic infiltration, IgG4-positive plasma cells infiltration, storiform fibrosis, and obliterative phlebitis. IgG4-RD can affect multiple organs or tissues, such as the hypophysis pituitary gland, lacrimal gland, submandibular gland, thyroid, lung, pancreas, bile duct, kidney, retroperitoneal tissue, and prostate, resulting in swelling and sclerosis of the involved organs (Uchida et al. 2016). However, the specific role of IgG4 is still remains unclear.

The history of research and discovery IgG4-RD is provided in detail in another chapter. Although IgG4-RD is the general name given to the overall condition, several names have been put forward to describe this entity. In 2001, IgG4-RD was first identified in the context to the pancreas and was termed "sclerosing pancreatitis," which is now referred to as type I autoimmune pancreatitis (AIP) (Hamano et al. 2001). Previous to this, Yoshida et al. (1995) firstly described AIP based on patients that showed a diffusely enlarged pancreas, a narrowing main pancreatic duct, increased serum IgG levels, the presence of autoantibodies, fibrotic changes with lymphocytic infiltration, and steroidal efficacy. Thus, sclerosing pancreatitis can be considered to be synonymous with AIP.

AIP is often complicated by extra-pancreatic lesion with involvement of other organ and is therefore now considered as systemic disease rather than as a pancreas-specific disease. Accordingly, Kamisawa et al. (2006) proposed IgG4-related sclerosing disease. Similarly, Yamamoto et al. (2006) coined the term as "IgG4-related plasmacytic disease" from the perspective of Mikulicz's disease (Yamamoto et al. 2006). The term "IgG4-related multiorgan lymphoproliferative syndrome" was also proposed by Masaki et al. (2009) for case involving a lymphoproliferative disorder. Based on these related concepts, the disease name has been recently unified under the umberella term of "IgG4-RD" (Umehara et al. 2012a, b).

AIP is currently classified into type 1 and type 2 following the International Consensus Diagnostic Criteria for Autoimmune Pancreatitis (ICDC) (Shimosegawa et al. 2011). Type 1AIP is recognized as a component of the pancreatic manifestation of IgG4-RD. Type2 AIP histologically shows neutrophilic infiltration within the lumen and epithelium of the interlobular ducts and is remarkably distinct from type 1 AIP.

Recently, the role of several cell types in regulatory capacities has become recognized, including interleukin (IL)-10-producing B cells (Mizoguchi et al. 2002), T cells (Groux et al. 1997), dendritic cells (DCs) (Fujita et al. 2006; Hoshino et al. 2011), and macrophages (Murai et al. 2009). IL-10 is a major immunosuppressive cytokine that was firstly discovered as a secreted cytokine from Th2 cells, which inhibits cytokine secretion by activated Th1 cells (Moore et al. 1990). It is generally considered that the pathogenesis of several immune-related diseases is linked to dysfunction in regulatory immune mechanisms. Indeed, the body of literature reporting new subsets of regulatory cells has been conducted in humans and animal models in recent years. Regulatory T cells (Tregs) and B cells (Bregs) are prime examples of immune regulatory cells. Here, we review the role of Tregs and Bregs in IgG4-RD.

2 Tregs

Human Tregs were first isolated from the peripheral blood and were characterized as $CD4^{+}CD25^{high}$ T cells by several independent groups in 2001 (Baecher-Allan et al. 2001; Dieckmann et al. 2001; Jonuleit et al. 2001; Levings et al. 2001), based on the finding in 1995 that mouse Tregs constitutively express CD25 (the interleukin-2 (IL-2) receptor α-chain) (Sakaguchi et al. 1995). Tregs express the transcription factor forkhead box P3 (Foxp3) is a key regulator gene for their development of Tregs (Hori et al. 2003; Fontenot et al. 2003; Khattri et al. 2003). Foxp3 is a member of the winged helix/forkhead family of transcription factors and was identified because its mutations caused early onsets of fatal autoimmune first diseases, which are now collectively called immunodysregulation, polyendocrinopathy, and enteropathy, X-linked (IPEX) syndrome, in mice and human (Katoh et al. 2013). Most of the $Foxp3^{+}$ Tregs are $CD4^{+}$ T cells that strongly express CD25, which can suppress the activation, proliferation, and function of immune cells, including $CD4^{+}$ and $CD8^{+}$ T cells, natural killer (NK) and NKT cells, B cells and antigen-presenting cells both in vitro and in vivo (Morikawa and Sakaguchi 2014). Depending on the type of Tregs considered, suppression is mainly carried out through cell/cell contact-dependent mechanisms (e.g., glucocorticoid-induced TNFR-related protein (GITR), cytotoxic T lymphocyte antigen 4 (CTLA-4), granzymes), the release of suppressive cytokines (e.g., transforming growth factor-beta (TGF-β) or IL-10), or the generation of suppressive metabolites (e.g., adenosine) (Sakaguchi et al. 2008a; Roncarolo et al. 2006; Sakaguchi et al. 2010). This unique ability enables Foxp3$^+$ Tregs to effectively control immune responses for preventing the development of autoimmune disease, immunopathology, and allergy, as well as to maintain allograft tolerance and fetal–maternal tolerance during pregnancy (Baecher-Allan and Hafler 2006; Buckner 2010).

Reduced levels of circulating CD4$^+$CD25^{high} Tregs have been identified in patients with several types of immune-related disease, specifically in individuals with juvenile idiopathic arthritis (de Kleer et al. 2004; Cao et al. 2004), psoriatic arthritis (Cao et al. 2004), hepatitis C virus-associated mixed cryoglobulinemia (Boyer et al. 2004), autoimmune liver disease (Longhi et al. 2004), systemic lupus erythematosus (SLE) (Liu et al. 2004; Crispin et al. 2003), and Kawasaki disease (Furuno et al. 2004). However, no significant difference has been detected in the numbers of CD4$^+$CD25^{high} Tregs between healthy control subjects and patients with spondyloarthritis (Cao et al. 2004), multiple sclerosis (Putheti et al. 2004; Viglietta et al. 2004), or immune-mediated type I diabetes (Lindley et al. 2005; Putnam et al. 2005). Increased numbers of circulating CD4$^+$CD25^{high} Tregs were observed in patients with primary Sjögren's syndrome (SS) (Gottenberg et al. 2005). Conflicting results have been reported for the role of peripheral CD4$^+$CD25^{high} Tregs in myasthenia graves (Balandina et al. 2005; Fattorossi et al. 2005), rheumatoid arthritis (RA) (Cao et al. 2003, 2004; Liu et al. 2004; van Amelsfort et al. 2004; Ehrenstein et al. 2004, Möttönen et al. 2005; Vigna-Pérez et al. 2005), and inflammatory bowel disease (Maul et al. 2005), with either decreased or similar levels observed in patients compared to healthy controls. Thus, reduced numbers of circulating CD4$^+$CD25^{high} Tregs is not a general feature in patients with immune-related diseases, nor are these cells necessarily reflective of the actual situation at the site of inflammation. Nevertheless, the common findings of the increased numbers of Tregs in several of these conditions suggest that the reason for failed regulation in the inflamed tissue may be insufficient or defective Tregs function due to either cell-intrinsic or cell-extrinsic factors. However, the precise mechanism remains unclear.

2.1 Subtypes of Tregs

Tregs were originally identified as thymus-derived cells (Sakaguchi et al. 1995). Recent studies have demonstrated that Tregs can further subdivided into distinct subsets, providing a partial explanation for the vast functional heterogeneity of these cells. Two major pathways have been identified to be related to Treg development. Differentiation of thymic-derived Tregs depends on high-affinity interactions with self-peptide/major histocompatibility complex (MHC) class II complexes during T cell development in the thymus, whereas peripheral-derived

Tregs develop in the periphery from naïve T cell precursors that upregulate Foxp3 expression when activated by foreign antigens in tolerogenic conditions. These subtypes are also known as natural Tregs (nTregs) and inducible Tregs, (iTregs), respectively, (Wing and Sakaguchi 2010; Littman and Rudensky 2010; Campbell and Koch 2011; Feuerer et al. 2009). Several Treg subsets have been described according to the differential expression of surface markers such as CD45RA, CD45RO, CD127, CCR6, CCR7, HLA-DR, CD39, CD95, ICOS, CD147, CD31, CD44, and/or CD62L (Darrasse-Jèze et al. 2005; Seddiki et al. 2006; Kleinewietfeld et al. 2005; Borsellino et al. 2007; Baecher-Allan et al. 2006; Haas et al. 2007; Fritzsching et al. 2006; Solstad et al. 2011; Ito et al. 2008; Smigiel et al. 2014).

$CD4^+$ T cell differentiation into the conventional T cell and Treg lineages can be identified according to specific phenotypic markers. All T cell lineages originate in the thymus and emigrate as naïve $CD45RA^+$ T cells, and the subsequent activation of naïve T cells in the periphery induces their differentiation into both conventional and regulatory subsets. Conventional T cells further differentiate into memory T cells, which can be reactivated. Two independent research groups reported the presence of $CD45RA^+$ Tregs in humans (Seddiki et al. 2006; Fritzsching et al. 2006). Human $CD45RA^+$ naïve Tregs also differentiate into $CD45RA^-$ effector Tregs. Effector Tregs are presumably induced from naïve Tregs after antigen contact in a specific context and appear to resemble a Treg population that exerts its suppressive function directly in inflamed tissues. For this reason, effector Tregs are equipped with homing and chemokine receptors as well as specific effector functions. In contrast, naïve Tregs appear to primarily function in secondary lymphoid tissues (Sakaguchi et al. 2008a). $CD45RA^-$ peripheral Treg compartments are converted to Treg-like cells, which are derived from conventional T cells. These converted Treg-like cells have cell surface marker expression similar to that thymus-derived Tregs (Miyara et al. 2009; Sakaguchi et al. 2010).

The effector Tregs subsets are heterogeneous with respect to the expression of inducible co-stimulatory molecules (ICOS). In the periphery, two functionally different subsets of effector Tregs, $ICOS^+$ or $ICOS^-$ effector Tregs, actively produce the suppressive cytokine IL-10 or TGF-β, respectively, (Ito et al. 2008). It has been reported that the growth of Tregs secreting IL-10 required DCs expressing high levels ICOS-ligand, as cell growth was prevent by blockade of ICOS–ICOS ligand signaling (Akbari et al. 2002). DCs play an important role in the proliferation of $ICOS^+$ or $ICOS^-$ Tregs. Activated plasmacytoid DCs (pDCs) preferentially promote the proliferation of the $ICOS^+$ Tregs through ICOS-ligand, whereas activated conventional DCs (cDCs) preferentially promote the proliferation of the autologous $ICOS^-$ Tregs through B7 signaling (Ito et al. 2008). Despite the vast amount of information on Tregs that has accumulated to date, research in this field is still ongoing, and it is expected that new subsets of Tregs will continue to be discovered.

2.2 Tregs in IgG4-RD

2.2.1 Circulating Tregs in Peripheral Blood in the Patient with IgG4-RD

There are few reports about the role of circulating Tregs in the development and progression of IgG4-RD. Miyoshi et al. (2008) attempted to clarify the role of Tregs in IgG4-RD and examined a Treg phenotype related to $CD4^{+}CD25^{high}$ and $CD4^{+}CD25^{+}CD45RA^{+}$ (naïve) expression in the peripheral blood of patients with type 1 AIP using flow cytometry. For comparison, patients with other pancreatic disease (idiopathic or alcoholic pancreatitis) and healthy subjects were analyzed as controls. In type 1 AIP patients, the proportion of circulatory naïve ($CD45RA^{+}$) Tregs was significantly decreased in the peripheral blood, whereas the major population of effector ($CD45RA^{-}$) Tregs was significantly increased. In a group of patients with untreated type 1 AIP, the number of $CD4^{+}CD25^{high}$ Tregs was positively correlated with serum levels of IgG4, whereas no such correlation was observed in the other groups. Furthermore, there was no significant correlation among Tregs phenotypes and immunologic marker other than serum IgG4 (Miyoshi et al. 2008). In addition, Kusuda et al. (2011) analyzed the proportion of $ICOS^{+}$ Tregs and IL-10^{+} Tregs in the peripheral blood of type 1 AIP patients, patients with other pancreatic disease, and healthy controls using flow cytometry. The ratio of $ICOS^{+}$ Tregs was significantly higher in the type 1 AIP patients than in the other two groups. The ratio of IL-10^{+} Tregs was also significantly higher in type 1 AIP patients than in the healthy control group. These findings suggest that a decrease in the number of naïve Tregs may be involved in the pathogenesis of type 1 AIP. Inducible Tregs may increase as a natural response against inflammation. Moreover, an increased number of $ICOS^{+}$ Tregs may promote IgG4 production via IL-10. On the other side, $ICOS^{-}$ Tregs may be involved in fibrosis via TGF-β.

2.2.2 Tregs in Involved Organ with IgG4-RD

Zen et al. (2007) reported that Th2 immune balance, regulatory cytokines, and $Foxp3^{+}$ Tregs play an important role in IgG4-related sclerosing pancreatitis (type 1 AIP) and cholangitis [IgG4-related sclerosing cholangitis (SC)]. IgG4-SC recognized as a disease entity characterized by sclerosing inflammation with abundant IgG4-positive plasma cells and was associated with type 1 AIP was associated in some cases. The authors examined gene expression patterns and conducted immunohistochemical analysis of several cytokines in the different patients groups. In patients with type 1 AIP and IgG4-SC, and extra-pancreatobiliary lesions [IgG4-dacryoadenitis and sialadenitis (DS)], the relative gene expression levels of IL-4, IL-10 and TGF-β were all significantly higher than those in patients with primary sclerosing cholangitis (PSC) and primary biliary cholangitis (PBC). $CD4^{+}CD25^{+}Foxp3^{+}$ Tregs frequently showed infiltration in type 1 AIP and

IgG4-SC, whereas such infiltration was rarely observed in patients with PSC and other disease controls. It has also been reported that the ratio of Foxp3-positive cells to infiltrated mononuclear cells (Foxp3/Mono) was significantly higher in the pancreas of patients with type 1 AIP compared to that in patients with alcoholic chronic pancreatitis (CP); moreover, the Foxp3/Mono and IgG4/Mono ratios were positively correlated (Kusuda et al. 2011). Koyabu et al. (2010) compared the laboratory and immunohistochemical findings of the liver biopsy specimens in the patients with IgG4-SC and PSC, and specifically determined the ratio of IgG4-, IgG1-, and Foxp3-positive cells to infiltrated mononuclear cells among specimens. The ratio of IgG4/G1-positive plasma cells was significantly higher in the livers of IgG4-SC patients than those of PSC patients. Similarly, the Foxp3/Mono ratio in patients with IgG4-SC was significantly increased compared with that of the PSC patients. Moreover, in the patients with IgG4-SC, Foxp3-positive cells were significantly correlated with IgG4-positive cells, whereas no such correlation was observed in the other groups. Based on the findings of these studies, it appears that the pattern of infiltrated Tregs parallels that of circulating Tregs.

Tanaka et al. (2012) reported Tregs and Th1/Th2 cytokine in Mikulicz's disease (IgG4-related sialadenitis) using immunohistochemistry and mRNA expression analysis. They found lymphocyte infiltration of various subsets in the labial salivary glands (LSGs) of SS patients, and the selective infiltration of IgG4-positive plasma cells and Tregs in the LSGs of patients with Mikulicz's disease (IgG4-related sialadenitis) patients. The mRNA expression levels for both Th1 and Th2 cytokines and chemokines in LSGs from patients with SS were significantly higher than those of controls, whereas the expression levels of both Th2 and Tregs were significantly higher in the patients with Mikulicz's disease than in controls. Furthermore, the expression of IL-4 or IL-10 in the LSGs was correlated with the IgG4:IgG ratio. In combination with the results of Zen's report mentioned above, these findings indicate that the Th2 microenvironment of the involved organ may play an important role in the development of IgG-4-RD.

There are two reports about the role of Tregs in IgG4-related kidney disease (RKD). Mizushima et al. (2012) analyzed the histological differentiation (including Tregs) in patients with IgG4-related tubulointerstitial nephritis (TIN) before and after steroid treatment. Before steroid therapy, common characterized included TIN-like dense lymphoplasmacytic infiltration, interstitial fibrosis, IgG4-positive plasma cells, $CD4^{+}CD25^{+}$ T cells, and $Foxp3^{+}$ cells infiltration. However, after steroid therapy, the lymphoplasmacytic infiltrated area decreased and regional fibrosis became evident in the renal interstitium. The number of IgG4-positive plasma cells and $Foxp3^{+}$ cells significantly decreased, even in the early stage of therapy, whereas $CD4^{+}$ or $CD8^{+}$ T cells continued to infiltrate to a certain degree in sites of persistent inflammation persisted in the later stage. The other report of Tregs in IgG4-RKD focused on the role of IgG4 production and fibrosis (Kawamura et al. 2015). In this study, interstitial lymphoplasmacytic and eosinophilic infiltration and the severity of interstitial fibrosis were more intense in IgG4-RKD patients than in patients with kidney lesions with SS and idiopathic TIN (ITIN). In terms of the Th1/Th2 balance, the ratio of $CXCR3^{+}/CD3^{+}$ (Th1) cells was higher in SS as compared with that in IgG4-RKD and ITIN. By contrast, the ratio of $CCR4^+/CD3^+$ (Th2) cells was not different among patients with the three diseases. The ratio of interstitial $IgG4^+/IgG^+$ plasma cells, $Foxp3^+/CD3^+$ cells, and TGF-$\beta1^+$ cells to the total number of infiltrated cells was higher in IgG4-RKD than in SS and ITIN. In IgG4-RD, there was a positive correlation between the ratio of $Foxp3^+/CD3^+$ cells and that of $IgG4^+/IgG^+$. In addition, there was a significant correlation between the ratio of $Foxp3^+/CD3^+$ cells and that of TGF-$\beta1^+$ cells to the total number of infiltrating cells in IgG4-RKD. Furthermore, $Foxp3^+$ cells and TGF-$\beta1^+$ cells were co-localized in the interstitium in IgG4-RKD. The ratio of TGF-$\beta1^+$ cells to total infiltrated cells also significantly correlated with the severity of fibrosis was noticed in IgG4-RKD patients. Moreover, the interstitial distribution of type III and type IV collagen was denser in IgG4-RKD than in SS. From these data, the authors concluded that in IgG4-RKD, Tregs may promote IgG4 production in the interstitium and the increase in TGF-β1 via Tregs may play a role in the interstitial fibrosis including type III and type IV collagens. Indeed, a substantial amount of Treg infiltration has been observed in the kidneys of patients with IgG4-RD compared with disease control as well as in patients with other forms of IgG4-RD.

Taken together, these reports about the role of Tregs in IgG4-RD have clearly demonstrated that the disease is associated with substantial Tregs infiltration, in the target organs. In addition, IL-10 producing Tregs might be linked to the promotion of IgG4 production. Moreover, TGF-β producing Tregs might play a role in fibrosis.

2.2.3 Functional Disorders of Treg in IgG4-RD

The findings of the studies summarized in the section above raise the question as to why inflammation is not efficiently suppressed in IgG4-RD in spite of the augmentation of Tregs at localized site. Two possible explanations are the severity of inflammation is too extreme for the Tregs to overcome, or that Treg function is negatively affected in these conditions. From the viewpoint of the Treg dysfunction, some interesting findings related to the role of mammalian sterile 20-like kinase-1 MST1/Mst1 have emerged in humans and animal models. Mst1 is a serine/threonine kinase that is known to play important roles in the control of immune cell trafficking, proliferation, and differentiation. Moreover, Mst1 was shown to be required for thymocyte selection and was particularly crucial for maintaining the function of Tregs (Ueda et al. 2012). Tomiyama et al. (2013) demonstrated that the Mst1 kinase plays a critical role in maintaining the suppressor function of Tregs through regulation of cell contact-dependent regulatory processes. They further demonstrated that $Mst1^{-/-}$ Tregs failed to prevent the development of experimental colitis and antigen-specific suppression of the proliferation of naïve T cells proliferation in mice indicating that knockout of this gene led to the loss of function of Tregs. Fukuhara et al. (2015) examined the methylation levels of CpG sites in the 5′ promoter region of *MST1* and the expression levels of *MST1* in Tregs from patients with type 1 AIP. They found that the number of CpG methylation sites in the 5′ region of *MST1* was increased in type 1 AIP patients with extrapancreatic lesions, whereas the methylation levels of AIP patients without extrapancreatic lesions were similar to those of controls. This increased frequency of methylated CpG sites was correlated with the number of affected extrapancreatic organs. Furthermore, the expression of *MST1* was significantly downregulated in the Tregs of type 1 AIP patients compared to those of controls. These results suggest that the decreased expression of *MST1* in Tregs from type 1 AIP patients due to hypermethylation of the promoter contributes to the pathological mechanism driving systemic IgG4-RD.

3 Bregs

The fundamental role of Bregs in suppressing pathological immune responses has been widely recognized (Mauri and Bosma 2012). The first study demonstrating that B cells are likely to play an immunoregulatory role was conducted in B cell-deficient (μMT) mice that were unable to recover from experimental autoimmune encephalitis (Wolf et al. 1996). Mizoguchi et al. (2002), who first proposed the term "regulatory B cells," reported the existence of a discrete population of IL-10-producing CD1d^{hi} Bregs that expanded with progression of chronic intestinal inflammatory in the mesenteric lymph nodes (Mizoguchi et al. 2002). Since IL-10 is key player in immunosuppressive mechanisms, most of the researchers on investigation of IL-10-producing B cell subsets.

After the first report of CD1d^{hi} Bregs, multiple subsets of IL-10-producing Bregs have been described in mice; including CD19^{+}CD21^{hi}CD23^{hi}CD24^{hi} transitional 2 marginal-zone precursor (T2-MZP) cells (Evans et al. 2007), CD5^{+}CD1d^{hi} B (B10) cells (Yanaba et al. 2008), CD19^{+}CD21^{hi}CD23^{-} marginal-zone (MZ) B cells (Gray et al. 2007), Tim-1+ B cells (Ding et al. 2011), CD138^{high} plasma cells (Shen et al. 2014), and CD138^{+}CD44^{hi} plasmablasts (Matsumoto et al. 2014).

Bregs also play an important role in the immune regulation in humans. Similar to mouse models, human Bregs are predominantly identified based on their ability to produce IL-10. To date, CD19^{+}CD24^{hi}CD38^{hi}CD1d^{hi} immature B cells (Blair et al. 2010) and CD19^{+}CD24^{hi}CD27^{+} B10 cells (Iwata et al. 2011), CD19^{+}CD38^{+}CD1d^{+}IgM^{+}CD147^{+} GrB^{+} B cells (Lindner et al. 2013), CD25^{hi}CD71^{hi}CD73^{lo} Br1 B cells (van de Veen et al. 2013), and CD19^{+}CD24^{hi}CD27^{int} plasamablasts (Matsumoto et al. 2014) have been identified as Bregs.

Human Bregs were described firstly as a CD19^{+}CD24^{hi}CD38^{hi} immature B cell population from healthy individuals and SLE patients in 2010 (Blair et al. 2010). CD19^{+}CD24^{hi}CD38^{hi} immature Bregs are considered to produce the highest amount of IL-10 among all B cell subsets populating the peripheral blood and, more importantly, are the only subset shown to suppress the differentiation and immune responses of both Th1 and Th17 cells. Moreover, CD19^{+}CD24^{hi}CD38^{hi} immature Bregs can also convert CD4^{+} T cells into Tregs (Flores-Borja et al. 2013).

Abnormality of CD19^{+}CD24^{hi}CD38^{hi} immature Bregs has been reported in several autoimmune diseases, including SLE and RA. Normally, CD19^{+}CD24^{hi}CD38^{hi}

immature Bregs suppress the differentiation of Th1 cells induced by CD40 stimulation via IL-10; however, $CD19^{+}CD24^{hi}CD38^{hi}$ immature Bregs from the peripheral blood of SLE patients were unable to suppress the Th1 response because of impaired IL-10 production following CD40 stimulation (Blair et al. 2010). Similarly, in patients with active RA, $CD19^{+}CD24^{hi}CD38^{hi}$ immature Bregs were unable to induce Tregs or suppress Th17 responses (Flores-Borja et al. 2013). Although primarily studied in the context of autoimmunity, immature Bregs have also been reported to participate in the immune reaction in infectious diseases and transplantation. For example, in patients with human immunodeficiency virus infection, the frequency of IL-10-producing $CD19^{+}CD24^{hi}CD38^{hi}$ immature Bregs correlated positively with the viral load (Siewe et al. 2013). Furthermore, $CD19^{+}CD24^{hi}CD38^{hi}$ immature Bregs showed reduced IL-10-producing ability in chronic graft-versus-host disease (cGVHD) patients, compared with patients without cGVHD and healthy donors (Khoder et al. 2014).

Recently, a population of IL-10-producing Bregs named B10 cells was discovered in the peripheral blood from healthy individuals, and in patients with RA, SLE, SS, autoimmune vesiculobullous skin disease, or multiple sclerosis. The majority of the B10 cells were found within the $CD19^{+}CD24^{hi}CD27^{+}$ B-cell subpopulation, which are able to negatively regulate monocyte cytokine production via IL-10 pathways (Iwata et al. 2011). In the context of tumor immunology, one study showed that granzyme B (GrB)-expressing B cells with a $CD19^{+}CD38^{+}CD1d^{+}IgM^{+}CD147^{+}$ phenotype infiltrate tumors and regulate T cell responses (Lindner et al. 2013). In terms of allergen tolerance, another subset of Bregs was identified and termed as B regulatory 1 (Br1) cells, which displayed a $CD25^{hi}CD71^{hi}CD73^{lo}$ phenotype (van de Veen et al. 2013). Therefore, it seems clear that there are several subsets of Bregs. A list of these subsets and their phenotypes is provided in Table 1. The main reason is that Bregs have been predominantly investigated from the perspective of IL-10 producing B cells is that there is no conclusive transcriptional regulator of Bregs that is equivalent to Foxp3 in Tregs. This situation has thus complicated the analysis of the role of Bregs in disease.

3.1 Bregs in IgG4-RD

There are a few reports examining Bregs in the context of IgG4-RD. The first such report examined Bregs in patients with type 1 AIP. Sumimoto et al. (2014) analyzed the Breg subtypes, $CD19^{+}CD24^{high}CD38^{high}$ (immature) and $CD19^{+}CD24^{high}CD27^{+}$ (B10) from the peripheral blood of patients with type 1 AIP using flow cytometry. $ICD19^{+}CD24^{high}CD38^{high}$ immature Bregs were significantly increased in the peripheral blood of type 1 AIP patients compared with patients with CP and pancreatic cancer and healthy controls. Furthermore, $CD19^{+}CD24^{high}CD27^{+}$ B10 cells of type 1 AIP patients were decreased compared to those of the other groups, although the difference was not statistically significant. The total numbers of IL-10-producing B cells were not significantly different between type1 AIP patients and healthy controls.

Table 1 Representative Bregs subtypes in mice and human

Subtype	Phenotype		Reference
	Mouse	Human	
T2-MZP B cells	$CD19^{+}CD21^{hi}$ $CD23^{hi}CD24^{hi}$		Evans et al. (2007)
MZ B cells	$CD19^{+}CD21^{hi}CD23$		Gray et al. (2007)
B10 cells	$CD1d^{hi}CD5^{+}$	$CD19^{+}CD24^{hi}CD27^{+}$	Yanaba et al. (2008); Iwata et al. (2011)
B-1a cells	$CD5^{+}$		O'Garra et al. (1992)
Plasmablasts	$CD138^{+}CD44^{hi}$	$CD19^{+}CD24^{hi}CD27^{int}$	Matsumoto et al. (2014)
Plasma cells	$CD138^{hi}$		Shen et al. (2014)
TIM-1+B cells	$TIM\text{-}1^{+}CD19^{+}$		Ding et al. (2011)
Immature cells		$CD19^{+}CD24^{hi}CD38^{hi}$	Blair et al. (2010)
GrB+B cells		$CD19^{+}CD38^{+}CD1d^{+}IgM^{+}CD147^{+}$	Lindner et al. (2013)
Br1 cells		$CD25^{hi}CD71^{hi}CD73^{lo}$	van de Veen et al. (2013)

However, in untreated type 1 AIP patients, the number of $CD19^{+}CD24^{high}CD38^{high}$ immature Bregs and IgG4 was not correlated to IgG4 levels, which differs from the findings for Tregs described above. These results suggest that $CD19^{+}CD24^{high}CD38^{high}$ immature Bregs increase reactively to suppress disease activity, which is consistent with the hypothesis that $CD19^{+}CD24^{high}CD27^{+}$ B10 cells might be involved in the development of type 1 AIP.

Lin et al. (2014) explored the relationship of Bregs in IgG4-RD in patients with IgG4-RD diagnosed according to comprehensive IgG4-RD diagnostic criteria established in 2011. Compared to patients with SS and healthy controls, IgG4-RD patients had a lower frequency of peripheral $CD19^{+}CD24^{hi}CD38^{hi}$ immature Bregs. Furthermore, $CD19^{+}CD24^{-}CD38^{hi}$ immature Bregs subsets were significantly higher in the peripheral B cells from IgG4-RD patients than in those of SS patients and healthy individuals, which correlated with serum IgG4 levels. To our knowledge, there is no report of $CD19^{+}CD24^{-}CD38^{hi}$ B cells in the peripheral blood. However, this B cell subset was identified in pre-germinal center (pre-GC) cells in the tonsils (Palanichamy et al. 2009). In addition, the expression of levels B cell activating factor (BAFF) receptor and CD40 on B cells were significantly lower in IgG4-RD patients compared with those in SS patients and healthy individuals (Lin et al. 2014). These patterns of $CD19^{+}CD24^{hi}CD38^{hi}$ immature Bregs are in contrast to the findings in type 1 AIP patients. However, the clinical and demographic characteristics of the patients with IgG4-RD in this study were not clarified. There is evidence that the profile (e.g., age, sex) of patients with head and neck lesions of

IgG4-RD, including IgG4-DS, differ from that of patients with other type of IgG4-RD (Zen and Nakanuma 2010; Yamamoto et al. 2015). Therefore, these conflicting results among studies may be caused by differences in the involved organ of IgG4-RD.

4 B Cell Depletion Therapy

Recently, it was reported that rituximab was effective for the treatment of IgG4-RD, even without concomitant glucocorticoid therapy (Khosroshahi et al. 2012; Carruthers et al. 2015). However, the mechanism underlying the beneficial effects of rituximab for IgG4-RD remains unclear. Several investigators have reported the influence of rituximab on Tregs. Rituximab is a mouse–human chimeric antibody specific for CD20 that induces B cell depletion via Fc receptor-mediated antibody-dependent cell cytotoxicity and complement-dependent cytotoxicity mechanisms. Rituximab treatment depletes $CD20^+$ naïve and memory B cells from the peripheral blood. However, it is less effective in depleting tissue-resident marginal-zone and germinal center B cells and does not affect long-lived plasma cells, which do not express CD20. Rituximab have been evaluated for the treatment of not only non-Hodgkin's lymphoma as well as several autoimmune diseases, including RA, SLE, type 1 diabetes, idiopathic thrombocytopenic purpura, pemphigus vulgaris, mixed cryoglobulinaemia vasculitis (MCV), multiple sclerosis, and others. Interestingly, two separate cohort studies of patients with SLE reported that the frequency of $CD4^+CD25^{hi}$ T cells in the peripheral blood was substantially increased after B cell depletion (Vigna-Perez et al. 2006; Vallerskog et al. 2007; Anolik et al. 2007), and these T cells also expressed Foxp3 (Vallerskog et al. 2007). Furthermore, the proportion of $CD4^+$ T cells spontaneously producing IL-10 or TGF-β was increased in the rituximab-responsive patients (Vigna-Perez et al. 2006). Increased mRNA expression levels of gene associated with Tregs, such as *CD25*, *FOXP3*, *CTLA4*, and *GITR*, were observed in the rituximab-responsive patients (Sfikakis et al. 2007). However, *FOXP3* mRNA levels remained low in patients with SLE who did not respond to rituximab therapy and declined to baseline levels in patients who relapsed (Sfikakis et al. 2007). With response to the direct effect of rituximab against Bregs, it is has been proposed that rituximab might promote the repopulation with $CD19^+CD24^{hi}CD38^{hi}$ immature Bregs to lead to remission, because a high ratio of immature/memory B cells has been associated with long-term remission (Mauri and Bosma 2012).

MCV patients treated with rituximab also showed changes in effector T cells and Tregs populations (Saadoum et al. 2008). Specifically, the frequency of $CD4^+CD25^+Foxp3^+$ Tregs increased in rituximab-responsive MCV patients but not in non-responder patients or patients who relapsed in less than one year (Saadoun et al. 2008). Although the specific influence of rituximab against Bregs is unknown, these data suggest that the elimination of clonal B cells by rituximab treatment not only curtails effector T cell responses, but also promotes the expansion of Treg populations (Lund and Randall 2010).

$CD19^+CD27^+CD20^-CD38^{hi}$ plasmablasts, which are largely $IgG4^+$, play an important role in IgG4-RD disease activity. The number of $CD19^+CD27^+CD38^{hi}$ plasmablasts was found to decrease sharply after rituximab treatment, and the mechanism was attributed to depletion of $CD20^+$ precursors, since $CD19^+CD27^+CD38^{hi}$ plasmablasts do not express CD20 (Mattoo et al. 2014; Wallace et al. 2015).

Thus, further study is needed to comprehensively to analysis the mechanism underlying the effectiveness of rituximab in IgG4-RD, with specific focus on its influence on Tregs and Bregs.

5 Animal Models of Type 1 AIP

There are some animal models available for studying diseases related Treg depletion or dysfunction. Neonatal thymectomy (nTx) in certain mouse strains is known to induce organ-specific autoimmunity due to the disappearance of the supply of Tregs from the thymus. The depletion of Tregs then initiates an autoimmune response from peripheral tolerance (Sakaguchi et al. 1995). Thus, nTx mice have been used to establish an accurate animal model to mimic human type 1 AIP. Several autoantibodies have been associated with type 1 AIP. Anti-lactoferrin (LF) antibody was detected of 73.1 % patients with type 1 AIP, anti nuclear antibody (ANA) was detected in 69.2 % of patients, anti-carbonic anhydrase (CA)-II was detected in 53.8 %, rheumatoid factor was detected in 23.1 %, anti-smooth muscle antibody was detected in 15.4 %, anti-glutamic acid decarboxylase antibody was detected in 3.8 %, and anti-islet cell antibody was detected in 3.8 %. However, AMA was not found in the sera of any of these patients (Asada et al. 2006). The authors hypothesized that LF or CA-II may be candidates of target antigen in type 1 AIP and established animal models using nTx mice immunized with CA-II or LF. These mice showed lymphoplasmacytic infiltration in the pancreas, salivary gland, and around the bile duct, which is are similar characteristics to human IgG4-RD (Uchida et al. 2002).

WBN/Kob rats spontaneously develop sialadenitis, thyroiditis, sclerotic cholangitis, and tubulointestinal nephritis because of congenitally decreased peripheral Tregs. In this model, $CD8^+$ T cells seem to be effector cells although the target antigens are unknown. WBN/Kob rats showed deposition of tissue-specific IgG2b in the injured pancreas and lachrymal glands (Sakaguchi et al. 2008b). Although details of the IgG subclass in rodents remain unclear, rat IgG2b, a minor subclass of IgG, is separated to a similar position as human IgG4 by electrophoresis, indicating potentially similar roles. Thus, these animal models are useful for exploring the effect of the absence or decreased number of Tregs on the development of systemic inflammation.

From the perspective of Tregs function, another animal model has been established based on depletion of *Mst1*. *Mst1*-deficient mice spontaneously developed inflammatory infiltrates in multiple organs that increased with age and were accompanied by autoantibodies. One-year-old $Mst1^{-/-}$mice exhibited lymphoplasamcytic infiltration in the liver, lung, pancreas, and kidney, similar to IgG4-RD (Ueda et al. 2012). As described above, $Mst1^{-/-}$ Tregs loss their regulatory function. Therefore, $Mst1^{-/-}$mice cannot prevent the autoimmune reaction (Tomiyama et al. 2013).

In humans, it is well known that Tregs are increased in affected organs, and it is thought that these increased Tregs may be inducible Tregs. Observation of MRL/Mp mice treated with poly I:C support this speculation. An MRL/Mp mouse spontaneously develops severe autoimmune diseases such as glomerulonephritis, arteritis, sialadenitis, and arthritis, associated with autoantibodies. Yamashina et al. (2012) reported that poly I:C-treated MRL/Mp mice developed inflammatory cell infiltrates with acinar cell destruction and replacement by fibrous tissues, as observed in type 1 AIP. They further explored the effects of different models of administration of poly I:C in three strains of mice (MRL/Mp, BALB/c, and C57BL/6) and in three mouse models of pancreatitis without an autoimmune mechanism (cerulein-, pancreatic duct ligation-, and ligation+cerulein-treated mice) by making a comparative study of the immunohistochemical features of the pancreas. These 3 mouse models can serve as models for acute (Cerulein-treated), chronic (Ligation-treated) and severe pancreatitis (Ligation+Cerulein-treated). In only the poly I:C-treated MRL/Mp mice, $FOXP3^+$ Tregs showed an abundant infiltration at the early stage of the immune-mediated pancreatitis (Koyabu et al. 2013). These findings imply that Tregs are infiltrated at the early stage and are thus involved in the development of type 1 AIP.

Overall, studies with animal models have suggested that Tregs might play an important role in the development of IgG4-RD via various mechanisms.

6 Our Hypothesis of the Pathophysiology of IgG4-RD

Based on the evidence accumulated to date and summarized herein, we can propose the following hypothesis for the pathophysiology of IgG4-RD. Decreased numbers of naïve regulatory T cells and $CD19^+CD24^{high}CD27^+$ regulatory B cells may be involved in the induction of IgG4-RD. Moreover, effector/inducible Tregs and $CD19^+CD24^+CD38^{high}$ B10 cells increase in a reactive manner. It is well known that Th2 immune responses promote disease progression. Thus, increased numbers of inducible Tregs and $CD19^+CD24^+CD38^{high}$ B10 cells may also support the development and progress of IgG4-RD. Both of innate and adaptive immunity may affect the production of IgG4 and fibrosis development. In adaptive immunity, ICOS-positive Tregs might regulate IgG4 production via secretion of IL-10. In

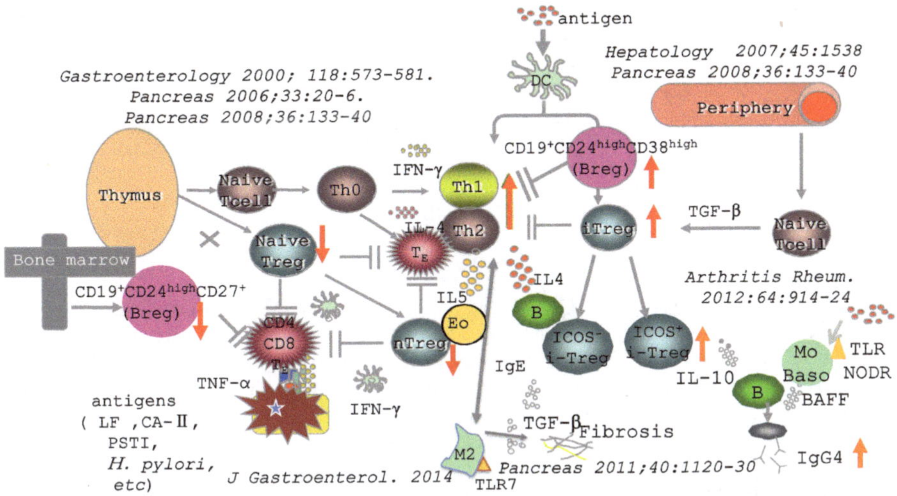

Fig. 1 Proposed hypothesis for the pathophysiology of type 1 AIP. Decreased numbers of naïve regulatory T cells (Tregs) and $CD19^+CD24^{high}CD27^+$ regulatory B cells (Bregs) may be involved in the induction of type 1 AIP. Inducible regulatory T cells (iTregs) and $CD19^+$ $CD24^+$ $CD38^{high}$ Bregs increased reactively. The progression of disease is then promoted by an increased Th2 immune response. The production of IgG4 may be regulated by IL-10 secreted from ICOS-positive Tregs and basophils and monocytes also regulate the production of IgG4 via TLR and NOD-like receptor signaling. Fibrosis may be regulated by TGF-β secreted from ICOS-negative Tregs and M2 macrophages. M2 macrophages may also contribute to the Th2 immune response in type 1 AIP. *AIP* autoimmune pancreatitis, *IgG4* immunoglobulin G4. *TLR* toll-like receptor, *NOD* nucleotide-binding oligomerization domain, ICOS inducible costimulator. The figure was reprinted from Okazaki K and Uchida K. Pancreas. 2015;44:1006–1016 with kind permission from Wolters Kluwer Health, Inc.

innate immunity, basophils and monocytes are also regulated via BAFF using TLR and nucleotide-binding oligomerization domain (NOD)-like receptor signaling pathway. Fibrosis may in turn be regulated by TGF-β secreted from ICOS-negative Tregs and M2 macrophage, which perform a suppressive function against inflammation. M2 macrophages also accelerate the Th2 immune response (Fig. 1).

7 Conclusion

In conclusion, Tregs and Bregs seem to be of critical importance to the pathogenesis of IgG4-RD. However, further studies are necessary to clarify the precise mechanism of immune regulation by Tregs and Bregs in IgG4-RD. When considered in the context of the effectiveness of rituximab, it will be worthy of note to elucidate the role of Tregs and Bregs in IgG4-RD.

Acknowledgments This study was partially supported by (1) JSPS KAKENHI Grant Numbers 26461038, 15K09052, and (2) a Grant-in-Aid for "Research for Intractable Diseases" Program from the Ministry of Labor and Welfare of Japan.

Figure 1 was reprinted from Pancreas, Okazaki K, Uchida K. Autoimmune Pancreatitis: The Past, Present, and Future. 1006–1613, 2015, with permission from Wolters Kluwer Health Inc.

References

Akbari O, Freeman GJ, Meyer EH, Greenfield EA, Chang TT, Sharpe AH, Berry G, DeKruyff RH, Umetsu DT (2002) Antigen-specific regulatory T cells develop via the ICOS-ICOS-ligand pathway and inhibit allergen-induced airway hyperreactivity. Nat Med 8(9):1024–1032

Anolik JH, Barnard J, Owen T, Zheng B, Kemshetti S, Looney RJ, Sanz I (2007) Delayed memory B cell recovery in peripheral blood and lymphoid tissue in systemic lupus erythematosus after B cell depletion therapy. Arthritis Rheum 56(9):3044

Asada M, Nishio A, Uchida K, Kido M, Ueno S, Uza N, Kiriya K, Inoue S, Kitamura H, Ohashi S, Tamaki H, Fukui T, Matsuura M, Kawasaki K, Nishi T, Watanabe N, Nakase H, Chiba T, Okazaki K (2006) Identification of a novel autoantibody against pancreatic secretory trypsin inhibitor in patients with autoimmune pancreatitis. Pancreas 33(1):20–26

Baecher-Allan C, Hafler DA (2006) Human regulatory T cells and their role in autoimmune disease. Immunol Rev 212:203–216

Baecher-Allan C, Brown JA, Freeman GJ, Hafler DA (2001) $CD4^{+}CD25$ high regulatory cells in human peripheral blood. J Immunol 167(3):1245–1253

Baecher-Allan C, Wolf E, Hafler DA (2006) MHC class II expression identifies functionally distinct human regulatory T cells. J Immunol 176(8):4622–4631

Balandina A, Lecart S, Dartevelle P, Saoudi A, Berrih-Aknin S (2005) Functional defect of regulatory $CD4^{+}CD25^{+}$ T cells in the thmus of patients with autoimmune Myasthenia Gravis. Blood 105(2):734–741

Blair PA, Noreña LY, Flores-Borja F, Rawlings DJ, Isenberg DA, Ehrenstein MR, Mauri C (2010) CD19(+)CD24(hi)CD38(hi) B cells exhibit regulatory capacity in healthy individuals but are functionally impaired in systemic lupus erythematosus patients. Immunity 32(1):129–140. doi:10.1016/j.immuni.2009.11.009

Borsellino G, Kleinewietfeld M, Di Mitri D, Sternjak A, Diamantini A, Giometto R, Höpner S, Centonze D, Bernardi G, Dell'Acqua ML, Rossini PM, Battistini L, Rötzschke O, Falk K (2007) Expression of ectonucleotidase CD39 by $Foxp3^{+}$ Treg cells: hydrolysis of extracellular ATP and immune suppression. Blood 110(4):1225–1232

Boyer O, Saadoun D, Abrio J, Dodille M, Piette JC, Cacoub P, Klatzmann D (2004) $CD4^{+}CD25^{+}$ regulatory T-cell deficiency in patients with hepatitis C-mixed cryoglobulinemia vasculitis. Blood 103(9):3428–3430

Buckner JH (2010) Mechanisms of impaired regulation by $CD4^{+}CD25^{+}FOXP3^{+}$ regulatory T cells in human autoimmune disease. Nat Rev Immunol 10(12):849–859

Campbell DJ, Koch MA (2011) Phenotypical and functional specialization of $FOXP3^{+}$ regulatory T cells. Nat Rev Immunol 11(2):119–130

Cao D, Malmstrom V, Baecher-Allan C, Klareskog L, Trollmo C (2003) Isolation and functional characterization of regulatory CD25 bright $CD4^{+}$ T cells from the target organ of patients with rheumatoid arthritis. Eur J Immunol 33(1):215–223

Cao D, van Vollenhoven R, Klareskog L, Trollmo C, Malmström V (2004) CD25 bright $CD4^{+}$ regulatory T cells are enriched in inflamed joints of patients with chronic rheumatic disease. Arthritis Res Ther 6(4):335–346

Carruthers MN, Topazian MD, Khosroshahi A, Witzig TE, Wallace ZS, Hart PA, Deshpande V, Smyrk TC, Chari S, Stone JH (2015) Rituximab for IgG4-related disease: a prospective, open-label trial. Ann Rheum Dis 74(6):1171–1177. doi:10.1136/annrheumdis-2014-206605

Crispin JC, Martinez A, Alcocer-Verela J (2003) Quantification of regulatory T cells in patients with systemic lupus erythematosus. J Autoimmun 21(3):273–276

Darrasse-Jèze G, Marodon G, Salomon BL, Catala M, Klatzmann D (2005) Ontogeny of $CD4^{+}CD25^{+}$ regulatory/suppressor T cells in human fetuses. Blood 105(12):4715–4721

de Kleer IM, Wedderburn LR, Taams LS, Patel A, Varsani H, Klein M, de Jager W, Pugayung G, Giannoni F, Rijkers G, Albani S, Kuis W, Prakken B (2004) CD4 CD25 bright regulatory T cells actively regulate inflammation in the joints of patients with the remitting from of juvenile idiopathic arthritis. J Iimunol 172(10):6435–6443

Dieckmann D, Plottner H, Berchtold S, Berger T, Schuler G (2001) Ex vivo isolation and characterization of CD4(+)CD25(+) T cells with regulatory properties from human blood. J Exp Med 193(11):1303–1310

Ding Q, Yeung M, Camirand G, Zeng Q, Akiba H, Yagita H, Chalasani G, Sayegh MH, Najafian N, Rothstein DM (2011) Regulatory B cells are identified by expression of TIM-1 and can be induced through TIM-1 ligation to promote tolerance in mice. J Clin Invest 121 (9):3645–3656. doi:10.1172/JCI46274

Ehrenstein MR, Evans JG, Singh A, Moore S, Warnes G, Isenberg DA, Mauri C (2004) Compromised function of regulatory T cells in rheumatoid arthritis and reversal by anti-TNF alpha therapy. J Exp Med 200(3):277–285

Evans JG, Chavez-Rueda KA, Eddaoudi A, Meyer-Bahlburg A, Rawlings DJ, Ehrenstein MR, Mauri C (2007) Novel suppressive function of transitional 2 B cells in experimental arthritis. J Immunol 178(12):7868–7878

Fattorossi A, Battaglia A, Buzzonetti A, Ciaraffa F, Scambia G, Evoli A (2005) Circulating and thymic $CD4^{+}CD25^{+}$ T regulatory cells in myasthenia gravis: effect of immunosuppressive treatment. Immunology 116(1):134–141

Feuerer M, Hill JA, Mathis D, Benoist C (2009) $Foxp3^{+}$ regulatory T cells: differentiation, specification, subphenotypes. Nat Immunol 10(7):689–695

Flores-Borja F, Bosma A, Ng D, Reddy V, Ehrenstein MR, Isenberg DA, Mauri C (2013) $CD19^{+}CD24^{hi}$ $CD38^{hi}$ B cells maintain regulatory T cells while limiting TH1 and TH17 differentiation. Sci Transl Med 5(173):173ra23. doi:10.1126/scitranslmed.3005407

Fontenot JD, Gavin MA, Rudensky AY (2003) Foxp3 programs the development and function of $CD4^{+}CD25^{+}$ regulatory T cells. Nat Immunol 4(4):330–336

Fritzsching B, Oberle N, Pauly E, Geffers R, Buer J, Poschl J, Krammer P, Linderkamp O, Suri-Payer E (2006) Naive regulatory T cells: a novel subpopulation defined by resistance toward CD95L-mediated cell death. Blood 108(10):3371–3378

Fujita S, Seino K, Sato K, Sato Y, Eizumi K, Yamashita N, Taniguchi M, Sato K (2006) Regulatory dendritic cells act as regulators of acute lethal systemic inflammatory response. Blood 107:3656–3664

Fukuhara T, Tomiyama T, Yasuda K, Ueda Y, Ozaki Y, Son Y, Nomura S, Uchida K, Okazaki K, Kinashi T (2015) Hypermethylation of MST1 in IgG4-related autoimmune pancreatitis and rheumatoid arthritis. Biochem Biophys Res Commun 463(4):968–974. doi:10.1016/j.bbrc.2015.06.043

Furuno K, Yuge T, Kusuhara K, Takada H, Nishio H, Khajoee V, Ohno T, Hara T (2004) $CD25^{+}CD4^{+}$ regulatory T cells in patients with Kawasaki disease. J Pediatr 145(3):385–390

Gottenberg JE, Lavie F, Abbed K, Gasnault J, Le Nevot E, Delfraissy JF, Taoufik Y, Mariette X (2005) CD4 CD25 high regulatory T cells are not impaired in patients with primary Sjogren's syndrome. J Autoimmun 24(3):235–242

Gray M, Miles K, Salter D, Gray D, Savill J (2007) Apoptotic cells protect mice from autoimmune inflammation by the induction of regulatory B cells. Proc Natl Acad Sci USA 104:14080–14085

Groux H, O'Garra A, Bigler M, Rouleau M, Antonenko S, de Vries JE, Roncarolo MG (1997) A $CD4^+$ T-cell subset inhibits antigen-specific T-cell responses and prevents colitis. Nature 389 (6652):737–742

Haas J, Fritzsching B, Trubswetter P, Korporal M, Milkova L, Fritz B, Vobis D, Krammer PH, Suri-Payer E, Wildemann B (2007) Prevalence of newly generated naive regulatory T cells (Treg) is critical for Treg suppressive function and determines Treg dysfunction in multiple sclerosis. J Immunol 179(2):1322–1330

Hamano H, Kawa S, Horiuchi A, Unno H, Furuya N, Akamatsu T, Fukushima M, Nikaido T, Nakayama K, Usuda N, Kiyosawa K (2001) High serum IgG4 concentrations in patients with sclerosing pancreatitis. N Engl J Med 344(10):732–738

Hori S, Nomura T, Sakaguchi S (2003) Control of regulatory T cell development by the transcription factor Foxp3. Science 299(5609):1057–1061

Hoshino S, Kurishima A, Inaba M, Ando Y, Fukui T, Uchida K, Nishio A, Iwai H, Yokoi T, Ito T, Hasegawa-Ishii S, Shimada A, Li M, Okazaki K, Ikehara S (2011) Amelioration of 2,4,6-trinitrobenzene sulfonic acid-induced colitis in mice by immunoregulatory dendritic cells. J Gastroenterol 46:1368–1381

Ito T, Hanabuchi S, Wang YH, Park WR, Arima K, Bover L, Park WR, Arima K, Bover L, Qin FX, Gilliet M, Liu YJ (2008) Two functional subsets of $FOXP3^+$ regulatory T cells in human thymus and periphery. Immunity 28(6):870–880

Iwata Y, Matsushita T, Horikawa M, Dilillo DJ, Yanaba K, Venturi GM, Szabolcs PM, Bernstein SH, Magro CM, Williams AD, Hall RP, St Clair EW, Tedder TF (2011) Characterization of a rare IL-10-competent B-cell subset in humans that parallels mouse regulatory B10 cells. Blood 117(2):530–541. doi:10.1182/blood-2010-07-294249

Jonuleit H, Schmitt E, Stassen M, Tuettenberg A, Knop J, Enk AH (2001) Identification and functional characterization of human CD4(+)CD25(+) T cells with regulatory properties isolated from peripheral blood. J Exp Med 193(11):1285–1294

Kamisawa T, Nakajima H, Egawa N, Funata N, Tsuruta K, Okamoto A (2006) IgG4-related sclerosing disease incorporating sclerosing pancreatitis, cholangitis, sialadenitis and retroperitoneal fibrosis with lymphadenopathy. Pancreatology. 6(1–2):132–137

Katoh H, Zheng P, Liu Y (2013) FOXP3: genetic and epigenetic implications for autoimmunity. J Autoimmun 41:72–78. doi:10.1016/j.jaut.2012.12.004

Kawamura E, Hisano S, Nakashima H, Takeshita M, Saito T (2015) Immunohistological analysis for immunological response and mechanism of interstitial fibrosis in IgG4-related kidney disease. Mod Rheumatol 25(4):571–578. doi:10.3109/14397595.2014.1001474

Khattri R, Cox T, Yasayko SA, Ramsdell F (2003) An essential role for Scurfin in $CD4^+CD25^+$ T regulatory cells. Nat Immunol 4(4):337–342

Khoder A, Sarvaria A, Alsuliman A et al (2014) Regulatory B cells are enriched within the IgM memory and transitional subsets in healthy donors but are deficient in chronic GVHD. Blood 124:2034

Khosroshahi A, Carruthers MN, Deshpande V, Unizony S, Bloch DB, Stone JH (2012) Rituximab for the treatment of IgG4-related disease: lessons from 10 consecutive patients. Med (Baltimore) 91(1):57–66. doi:10.1097/MD.0b013e3182431ef6

Kleinewietfeld M, Puentes F, Borsellino G, Battistini L, Rotzschke O, Falk K (2005) CCR6 expression defines regulatory effector/memory-like cells within the CD25(+)$CD4^+$ T-cell subset. Blood 105(7):2877–2886

Koyabu M, Uchida K, Miyoshi H, Sakaguchi Y, Fukui T, Ikeda H, Takaoka M, Hirohara J, Nishio A, Uemura Y, Uemoto S, Okazaki K (2010) Analysis of regulatory T cells and IgG4-positive plasma cells among patients of IgG4-related sclerosing cholangitis and autoimmune liver diseases. J Gastroenterol 45(7):732–741. doi:10.1007/s00535-010-0199-3

Koyabu M, Uchida K, Sakaguchi Y, Fukata N, Kusuda T, Miyoshi H, Yoshida K, Sumimoto K, Mitsuyama T, Fukui T, Nishio A, Okazaki K (2013) Possible involvement of Foxp3(+) regulatory T cells in the development of immune-mediated pancreatitis in MRL/Mp mice treated with polyinosinic: polycytidylic acid. Int J Rheumatol 2013:367–325. doi:10.1155/2013/367325

Kusuda T, Uchida K, Miyoshi H, Koyabu M, Satoi S, Takaoka M, Shikata N, Uemura Y, Okazaki K (2011) Involvement of inducible costimulator and interleukin 10-positive regulatory T cells in the development of IgG4-related autoimmune pancreatitis. Pancreas 40(7):1120–1130. doi:10.1097/MPA.0b013e31821fc796

Levings MK, Sangregorio R, Roncarolo MG (2001) Human CD25(+)CD4(+) T regulatory cells suppress naive and memory T cell proliferation and can be expanded in vitro without loss of function. J Exp Med 193:1295–1302

Lin W, Jin L, Chen H, Wu Q, Fei Y, Zheng W, Wang Q, Li P, Li Y, Zhang W, Zhao Y, Zeng X, Zhang F (2014) B cell subsets and dysfunction of regulatory B cells in IgG4-related diseases and primary Sjögren's syndrome: the similarities and differences. Arthritis Res Ther 29, 16(3): R118. doi:10.1186/ar4571

Lindley S, Dayan CM, Bishop A, Roep BO, Peakman M, Tree TI (2005) Defective suppressor function in CD4(+)CD25(+) T-cells from patients with type I diabetes. Diabetes 193(1):1303–1310

Lindner S, Dahlke K, Sontheimer K, Hagn M, Kaltenmeier C, Barth TF, Beyer T, Reister F, Fabricius D, Lotfi R, Lunov O, Nienhaus GU, Simmet T, Kreienberg R, Möller P, Schrezenmeier H, Jahrsdörfer B (2013) Interleukin 21-induced granzyme B-expressing B cells infiltrate tumors and regulate T cells. Cancer Res 73(8):2468–2479. doi:10.1158/0008-5472.CAN-12-3450

Littman DR, Rudensky AY (2010) Th17 and regulatory T cells in mediating and restraining inflammation. Cell 140(6):845–858

Liu MF, Wang CR, Fung LL, Wu CR (2004) Decreased $CD4^{+}CD25^{+}$ T cells in periferal blood of patients with systemic lupus erythematosus. Scand J Immunol 59(2):198–202

Longhi MS, Ma Y, Bogdanos DP, Cheeseman P, Mieli-Vergani G, Vergani D (2004) Impairment of $CD4^{+}CD25^{+}$ regulatory T cells in autoimmune liver disese. J Hepatol 41(1):31–37

Lund FE, Randall TD (2010) Effector and regulatory B cells: modulators of $CD4^{+}$ T cell immunity. Nat Rev Immunol 10(4):236–247. doi:10.1038/nri2729

Masaki Y, Dong L, Kurose N, Kitagawa K, Morikawa Y, Yamamoto M, Takahashi H, Shinomura Y, Imai K, Saeki T, Azumi A, Nakada S, Sugiyama E, Matsui S, Origuchi T, Nishiyama S, Nishimori I, Nojima T, Yamada K, Kawano M, Zen Y, Kaneko M, Miyazaki K, Tsubota K, Eguchi K, Tomoda K, Sawaki T, Kawanami T, Tanaka M, Fukushima T, Sugai S, Umehara H (2009) Proposal for a new clinical entity, IgG4-positive multiorgan lymphoproliferative syndrome: analysis of 64 cases of IgG4-related disorders. Ann Rheum Dis 68 (8):1310–1315. doi:10.1136/ard.2008.089169

Matsumoto M, Baba A, Yokota T, Nishikawa H, Ohkawa Y, Kayama H, Kallies A, Nutt SL, Sakaguchi S, Takeda K, Kurosaki T, Baba Y (2014) Interleukin-10-producing plasmablasts exert regulatory function in autoimmune inflammation. Immunity 41(6):1040–1051. doi:10.1016/j.immuni.2014.10.016

Mattoo H, Mahajan VS, Della-Torre E, Sekigami Y, Carruthers M, Wallace ZS, Deshpande V, Stone JH, Pillai S (2014) De novo oligoclonal expansions of circulating plasmablasts in active and relapsing IgG4-related disease. J Allergy Clin Immunol 134(3):679–687. doi:10.1016/j.jaci.2014.03.034

Maul J, Loddenkemper C, Mundt P, Berg E, Giese T, Stallmach A, Zeitz M, Duchmann R (2005) Peripheral and intestinal regulatory CD4+ CD25(high) T cells in inflammatory bowel disease. Gastroenterology 128(7):1868–1878

Mauri C, Bosma A (2012) Immune regulatory function of B cells. Annu Rev Immunol 30:221. doi:10.1146/annurev-immunol-020711-074934

Miyara M, Yoshioka Y, Kitoh A, Shima T, Wing K, Niwa A, Parizot C, Taflin C, Heike T, Valeyre D, Mathian A, Nakahata T, Yamaguchi T, Nomura T, Ono M, Amoura Z, Gorochov G, Sakaguchi S (2009) Functional delineation and differentiation dynamics of human $CD4^{+}$ T cells expressing the FoxP3 transcription factor. Immunity 30(6):899–911

Miyoshi H, Uchida K, Taniguchi T, Yazumi S, Matsushita M, Takaoka M, Okazaki K (2008) Circulating naïve and $CD4^{+}CD25$ high regulatory T cells in patients with autoimmune pancreatitis. Pancreas 36(2):133–140. doi:10.1097/MPA.0b013e3181577553

Mizoguchi A, Mizoguchi E, Takedatsu H, Blumberg RS, Bhan AK (2002) Chronic intestinal inflammatory condition generates IL-10-producing regulatory B cell subset characterized by CD1d upregulation. Immunity 16:219–230

Mizushima I, Yamada K, Fujii H, Inoue D, Umehara H, Yamagishi M, Yamaguchi Y, Nagata M, Matsumura M, Kawano M (2012) Clinical and histological changes associated with corticosteroid therapy in IgG4-related tubulointerstitial nephritis. Mod Rheumatol 22 (6):859–870. doi:10.1007/s10165-011-0589-2

Moore KW, Vieira P, Fiorentino DF, Trounstine ML, Khan TA, Mosmann TR (1990) Homology of cytokine synthesis inhibitory factor (IL-10) to the Epstein-Barr virus gene BCRFI. Science 248(4960):1230–1234

Morikawa H, Sakaguchi S (2014) Genetic and epigenetic basis of Treg cell development and function: from a FoxP3-centered view to an epigenome-defined view of natural Treg cells. Immunol Rev 259(1):192–205. doi:10.1111/imr.12174

Möttönen M, Heikkinen J, Mustonen I, Isomäki P, Luukkainen R, Lassila O (2005) $CD4^{+}CD25^{+}$ T cells with the phenotypic and functional characteristics of regulatory T cells are enriched in the synovial fluid of patients with rheumatoid arthritis. Clin Exp Immunol 140(2):360–367

Murai M, Turovskaya O, Kim G, Madan R, Karp CL, Cheroutre H, Kronenberg M (2009) Interleukin 10 acts on regulatory T cells to maintain expression of the transcription factor Foxp3 and suppressive function in mice with colitis. Nat Immunol 10(11):1178–1184. doi:10.1038/ni.1791

O'Garra A, Chang R, Go N, Hastings R, Haughton G, Howard M (1992) Ly-1 B (B-1) cells are the main source of B cell derived interleukin 10. Eur J Immunol 22(3):711–717

Palanichamy A, Barnard J, Zheng B, Owen T, Quach T, Wei C, Looney RJ, Sanz I, Anolik JH (2009) Novel human transitional B cell populations revealed by B cell depletion therapy. J Immunol 182(10):5982–5993. doi:10.4049/jimmunol.0801859

Putheti P, Pettersson A, Soderstrom M, Link H, Huang YM (2004) Circulating $CD4^{+}CD25^{+}$ T regulatory cells are not altered in multiple sclerosis and unaffected by disease-modulating drugs. J Clin Immunol 24(2):155–161

Putnam AL, Vendrame F, Dotta F, Gottlieb PA (2005) $CD4^{+}CD25$ high regulatory T cells in human autoimmune diabetes. J Autoimmun 24:55–62

Roncarolo MG, Gregori S, Battaglia M, Bacchetta R, Fleischhauer K, Levings MK (2006) Interleukin-10-secreting type 1 regulatory T cells in rodents and humans. Immunol Rev 212:28–50

Saadoun D, Rosenzwajg M, Landau D, Piette JC, Klatzmann D, Cacoub P (2008) Restoration of peripheral immune homeostasis after rituximab in mixed cryoglobulinemia vasculitis. Blood 111(11):5334–5341. doi:10.1182/blood-2007-11-122713

Sakaguchi S, Sakaguchi N, Asano M, Itoh M, Toda M (1995) Immunologic self-tolerance maintained by activated T cells expressing IL-2 receptor alpha-chains (CD25). Breakdown of a single mechanism of self-tolerance causes various autoimmune diseases. J Immunol 155 (3):1151–1164

Sakaguchi S, Yamaguchi T, Nomura T, Ono M (2008a) Regulatory T cells and immune tolerance. Cell 133(5):775–787. doi:10.1016/j.cell.2008.05.009

Sakaguchi Y, Inaba M, Tsuda M, Quan GK, Omae M, Ando Y, Uchida K, Okazaki K, Ikehara S (2008b) The Wistar Bonn Kobori rat, a unique animal model for autoimmune pancreatitis with extrapancreatic exocrinopathy. Clin Exp Immunol 152(1):1–12. doi:10.1111/j.1365-2249.2008.03588.x

Sakaguchi S, Miyara M, Costantino CM, Hafler DA (2010) $FOXP3^{+}$ regulatory T cells in the human immune system. Nat Rev Immunol 10(7):490–500. doi:10.1038/nri2785

Seddiki N, Santer-Nanan B, Tangye SG, Alexander SI, Solomon M, Lee S, Nanan R, de Saint Fazekas, Groth B (2006) Persistece of naïve $CD45RA^{+}$ regulatory T cells in adult life. Blood 107(7):2830–2838

Sfikakis PP, Souliotis VL, Fragiadaki KG, Moutsopoulos HM, Boletis JN, Theofilopoulos AN (2007) Increased expression of the FoxP3 functional marker of regulatory T cells following B cell depletion with rituximab in patients with lupus nephritis. Clin Immunol 23(1):66–73

Shen P, Roch T, Lampropoulou V, O'Connor RA, Stervbo U, Hilgenberg E, Ries S, Dang VD, Jaimes Y, Daridon C, Li R, Jouneau L, Boudinot P, Wilantri S, Sakwa I, Miyazaki Y, Leech MD, McPherson RC, Wirtz S, Neurath M, Hoehlig K, Meinl E, Grützkau A, Grün JR, Horn K, Kühl AA, Dörner T, Bar-Or A, Kaufmann SH, Anderton SM, Fillatreau S (2014) IL-35-producing B cells are critical regulators of immunity during autoimmune and infectious diseases. Nature 507(7492):366–370. doi:10.1038/nature12979

Shimosegawa T, Chari ST, Frulloni L, Kamisawa T, Kawa S, Mino-Kenudson M, Kim MH, Klöppel G, Lerch MM, Löhr M, Notohara K, Okazaki K, Schneider A, Zhang L, International Association of Pancreatology. (2011) International consensus diagnostic criteria for autoimmune pancreatitis: guidelines of the International Association of Pancreatology. Pancreas. 40 (3):352–8. doi:10.1097/MPA.0b013e3182142fd2

Siewe B, Stapleton JT, Martinson J, Keshavarzian A, Kazmi N, Demarais PM, French AL, Landay A (2013) Regulatory B cell frequency correlates with markers of HIV disease progression and attenuates anti-HIV $CD8^+$ T cell function in vitro. J Leukoc Biol 93(5):811–818. doi:10.1189/jlb.0912436

Smigiel KS, Richards E, Srivastava S, Thomas KR, Dudda JC, Klonowski KD, Campbell DJ (2014) CCR7 provides localized access to IL-2 and defines homeostatically distinct regulatory T cell subsets. J Exp Med 211(1):121–136

Solstad T, Bains SJ, Landskron J, Aandahl EM, Thiede B, Tasken K, Aandahl EM, Thiede B, Taskén K, Torgersen KM (2011) CD147 (Basigin/Emmprin) identifies $FoxP3^+CD45RO^+CTLA4^+$ activated human regulatory T cells. Blood 118(19):5141–5151

Sumimoto K, Uchida K, Kusuda T, Mitsuyama T, Sakaguchi Y, Fukui T, Matsushita M, Takaoka M, Nishio A, Okazaki K (2014) The role of $CD19^+CD24$ high CD38 high and $CD19^+CD24$ high $CD27^+$ regulatory B cells in patients with type 1 autoimmune pancreatitis. Pancreatology 14(3):193–200. doi:10.1016/j.pan.2014.02.004

Tanaka A, Moriyama M, Nakashima H, Miyake K, Hayashida JN, Maehara T, Shinozaki S, Kubo Y, Nakamura S (2012) Th2 and regulatory immune reactions contribute to IgG4 production and the initiation of Mikulicz disease. Arthritis Rheum 64(1):254–263. doi:10.1002/art.33320

Tomiyama T, Ueda Y, Katakai T, Kondo N, Okazaki K, Kinashi T (2013) Antigen-specific suppression and immunological synapse formation by regulatory T cells require the Mst1 kinase. PLoS ONE 8(9):e73874. doi:10.1371/journal.pone.0073874

Uchida K, Okazaki K, Nishi T, Uose S, Nakase H, Ohana M, Matsushima Y, Omori K, Chiba T (2002) Experimental immune-mediated pancreatitis in neonatally thymectomized mice immunized with carbonic anhydrase II and lactoferrin. Lab Invest 82(4):411–424

Uchida K, Miyoshi H, Ikeura T, Shimatani M, Takaoka M, Okazaki K (2016) Clinical and pathophysiological issues associated with type 1 autoimmune pancreatitis. Clin J Gastroenterol 9(1):7–12. doi:10.1007/s12328-016-0628-9

Ueda Y, Katagiri K, Tomiyama T, Yasuda K, Habiro K, Katakai T, Ikehara S, Matsumoto M, Kinashi T (2012) Mst1 regulates integrin-dependent thymocyte trafficking and antigen recognition in the thymus. Nat Commun 3:1098. doi:10.1038/ncomms2105

Umehara H, Okazaki K, Masaki Y, Kawano M, Yamamoto M, Saeki T, Matsui S, Sumida T, Mimori T, Tanaka Y, Tsubota K, Yoshino T, Kawa S, Suzuki R, Takegami T, Tomosugi N, Kurose N, Ishigaki Y, Azumi A, Kojima M, Nakamura S, Inoue D, Research Program for Intractable Disease by Ministry of Health, Labor and Welfare (MHLW) Japan G4 team (2012a) A novel clinical entity, IgG4-related disease (IgG4RD): general concept and details. Mod Rheumatol 22(1):1–14. doi:10.1007/s10165-011-0508-6

Umehara H, Okazaki K, Masaki Y, Kawano M, Yamamoto M, Saeki T, Matsui S, Yoshino T, Nakamura S, Kawa S, Hamano H, Kamisawa T, Shimosegawa T, Shimatsu A, Nakamura S, Ito T, Notohara K, Sumida T, Tanaka Y, Mimori T, Chiba T, Mishima M, Hibi T, Tsubouchi H, Inui K, Ohara H (2012b) Comprehensive diagnostic criteria for IgG4-related disease (IgG4-RD), 2011. Mod Rheumatol 22(1):21–30. doi:10.1007/s10165-011-0571-z

Vallerskog T, Gunnarsson I, Widhe M, Risselada A, Klareskog L, van Vollenhoven R, Malmström V, Trollmo C (2007) Treatment with rituximab affects both the cellular and the humoral arm of the immune system in patients with SLE. Clin Immunol 122(1):62–74

van Amelsfort JM, Jacobs KM, Bijlsma JW, Bijlsma JW, Lafeber FP, Taams LS (2004) $CD4^{+}CD25^{+}$ regulatory T cells in rheumatoid arthritis. Arthritis Rheum 50(9):2775–2785

van de Veen W, Stanic B, Yaman G, Wawrzyniak M, Söllner S, Akdis DG, Rückert B, Akdis CA, Akdis M (2013) IgG4 production is confined to human IL-10-producing regulatory B cells that suppress antigen-specific immune responses. J Allergy Clin Immunol 131(4):1204–1212. doi:10.1016/j.jaci.2013.01.014

Viglietta V, Baecher-Allan C, Weiner HL, Hafler DA (2004) Loss of functional suppression by $CD4^{+}CD25^{+}$ regulatory T patients with multiple sclerosis. J Exp Med 199(7):971–979

Vigna-Perez M, Hernández-Castro B, Paredes-Saharopulos O, Portales-Pérez D, Baranda L, Abud-Mendoza C, González-Amaro R (2006) Clinical and immunological effects of Rituximab in patients with lupus nephritis refractory to conventional therapy: a pilot study. Arthritis Res Ther 8(3):R83

Vigna-Pérez M, Abud-Mendoza C, Portillo-Salazar H, Alvarado-Sánchez B, Cuevas-Orta E, Moreno-Valdés R, Baranda L, Paredes-Saharopulos O, González-Amaro R (2005) Immune effects of therapy with adalimumab in patients with rheumatoid arthritis. Clin Exp Immunol 141(2):372–380

Wallace ZS, Deshpande V, Mattoo H, Mahajan VS, Kulikova M, Pillai S, Stone JH (2015) IgG4-related disease: clinical and laboratory features in one hundred twenty-five patients. Arthritis Rheumatol 67(9):2466–2475. doi:10.1002/art.39205

Wing K, Sakaguchi S (2010) Regulatory T cells exert checks and balances on self tolerance and autoimmunity. Nat Immunol 11(1):7–13

Wolf SD, Dittel BN, Hardardottir F, Janeway CA Jr (1996) Experimental autoimmune encephalomyelitis induction in genetically B cell-deficient mice. J Exp Med 184(6):2271

Yamamoto M, Takahashi H, Ohara M, Suzuki C, Naishiro Y, Yamamoto H, Shinomura Y, Imai K (2006) A new conceptualization for Mikulicz's disease as an IgG4-related plasmacytic disease. Mod Rheumatol 16(6):335–340

Yamamoto M, Yajima H, Takahashi H, Yokoyama Y, Ishigami K, Shimizu Y, Tabeya T, Suzuki C, Naishiro Y, Takano K, Yamashita K, Hashimoto M, Keira Y, Honda S, Abe T, Suzuki Y, Mukai M, Himi T, Hasegawa T, Imai K, Shinomura Y (2015) Everyday clinical practice in IgG4-related dacryoadenitis and/or sialadenitis: results from the SMART database. Mod Rheumatol 25(2):199–204. doi:10.3109/14397595.2014.950036

Yamashina M, Nishio A, Nakayama S, Okazaki T, Uchida K, Fukui T, Okazaki K (2012) Comparative study on experimental autoimmune pancreatitis and its extrapancreatic involvement in mice. Pancreas 41(8):1255–1262. doi:10.1097/MPA.0b013e31824a0e58

Yanaba K, Bouaziz JD, Haas KM, Poe JC, Fujimoto M, Tedder TF (2008) A regulatory B cell subset with a unique $CD1dhiCD5^{+}$ phenotype controls T cell-dependent inflammatory responses. Immunity 28(5):639–650. doi:10.1016/j.immuni.2008.03.017

Yoshida K, Toki F, Takeuchi T, Watanabe S, Shiratori K, Hayashi N (1995) Chronic pancreatitis caused by an autoimmune abnormality. Proposal of the concept of autoimmune pancreatitis. Dig Dis Sci 40(7):1561–1568

Zen Y, Nakanuma Y (2010) IgG4-related disease: a cross-sectional study of 114 cases. Am J Surg Pathol 34(12):1812–1819. doi:10.1097/PAS.0b013e3181f7266b

Zen Y, Fujii T, Harada K, Kawano M, Yamada K, Takahira M, Nakanuma Y (2007) Th2 and regulatory immune reactions are increased in immunoglobin G4-related sclerosing pancreatitis and cholangitis. Hepatology 45(6):1538–1546. doi:10.1002/hep.21697

IgG4-Related Disease and Innate Immunity

Tomohiro Watanabe, Kouhei Yamashita and Masatoshi Kudo

Abstract An increased number of clinicopathological studies on autoimmune pancreatitis, cholangitis, and sialoadenitis have led to the recognition of immunoglobulin G4-related disease (IgG4-RD) as a novel disorder, characterized by elevated levels of serum IgG4 and infiltration of IgG4-expressing plasma cells in the affected organs. Although the immunological background associated with the development of IgG4-RD remains poorly understood, recent studies have suggested involvement of the innate immune response in its pathogenesis. Peripheral blood innate immune cells, such as plasmacytoid dendritic cells and monocytes isolated from patients with IgG4-RD, promote IgG4 production by B cells. Activation of the innate immune response by microbe- and/or damage-associated molecular patterns stimulates production of type I interferon and B cell-activating factor by innate immune cells and results in IgG4 production by B cells. Elucidation of the innate immune response associated with IgG4-RD may help identify a new therapeutic target for this immune disorder.

Contents

T. Watanabe (✉) · M. Kudo
Department of Gastroenterology and Hepatology, Kindai University Faculty of Medicine, 377-2 Ohno-Higashi, Osaka-Sayama, Osaka 589-8511, Japan
e-mail: tmhrwtnb@kuhp.kyoto-u.ac.jp

K. Yamashita
Department of Hematology and Oncology, Kyoto University Graduate School of Medicine, Kyoto, Kyoto 606-8507, Japan

Current Topics in Microbiology and Immunology (2017) 401: 115–128
DOI 10.1007/82_2016_42

Published Online: 22 September 2016

1 Introduction

Immunoglobulin G4-related disease (IgG4-RD) is a chronic multiorgan fibroinflammatory disorder (Stone et al. 2012). It was first described by Japanese physicians and researchers who found elevated levels of serum IgG4 in most patients with autoimmune pancreatitis (AIP) (Hamano et al. 2001; Kamisawa and Okamoto 2006; Masaki et al. 2009; Okazaki et al. 2008). Physicians' awareness and recognition of IgG4-RD have expanded substantially, enabling gastroenterologists and clinical immunologists to establish specific diagnostic criteria. These include the presence of elevated serum IgG4, as well as the massive infiltration of IgG4-expressing plasmacytes in the affected organs (Stone et al. 2012). Various single-organ diseases, such as AIP, sialoadenitis, and retroperitoneal fibrosis, are now considered as organ-specific manifestations of systemic IgG4-RD, because they share an enhanced IgG4 response. Thus, our knowledge of the clinical and epidemiological features of IgG4-RD is expanding rapidly, and IgG4-RD is attracting increasing attention from gastroenterologists and clinical immunologists.

Although the clinical manifestations of IgG4-RD have been established in several organs, our understanding of its immune pathogenesis remains limited. Given the elevated IgG4 serum levels and abundant accumulation of IgG4-expressing plasmacytes in tissues, it is likely that adaptive immunity, rather than innate immunity, plays a pathogenic role in disease development. In fact, the remarkable efficacy of B cell depletion therapy (Carruthers et al. 2015; Khosroshahi et al. 2010) provides strong evidence that adaptive immune cells, such as B and T cells, are involved in the pathogenesis of IgG4-RD. In line with this, recent studies have suggested the involvement of abnormal adaptive immune responses, such as excessive T helper type 2 (TH2), regulatory T cells (Tregs), and plasmablasts (Mattoo et al. 2014b; Miyoshi et al. 2008; Satoguina et al. 2008; Wallace et al. 2015; Zen et al. 2007). However, these studies have not elucidated the abnormal immunological environment that leads to the development of IgG4-RD, and a number of unresolved questions have been raised. These include the identification of antigens recognized by elevated IgG4 levels and the pathogenicity of IgG4 itself. In addition, recent investigations have highlighted the importance of innate immunity in preceding and/or augmenting IgG4 responses driven by adaptive immunity (Akitake et al. 2010; Arai et al. 2015; Fukui et al. 2015; Watanabe et al. 2012, 2013). Thus, the cross talk between adaptive and innate immune responses is associated with the immune pathogenesis of IgG4-RD. In this review, we discuss the innate immune responses associated with IgG4-RD.

2 IgG4-Related Disease (IgG4-RD) and Microbe-Associated Molecular Patterns (MAMPs) and Damage-Associated Molecular Patterns (DAMPs)

2.1 *MAMPs and DAMPs*

Danger signals are initially recognized by the innate immune system, which then promotes antigen-specific adaptive immune responses. Innate immunity exerts its host–defense functions immediately upon recognition of microbe-associated molecular patterns (MAMPs) (Akira and Takeda 2004; Chen et al. 2009; Strober et al. 2006) and damage-associated molecular patterns (DAMPs) (Kono and Rock 2008), through germline-encoded pathogen recognition receptors (PRRs). In contrast, adaptive immunity is responsible for delayed effector functions, since it relies on the selection and clonal expansion of antigen-specific B cells and T cells via gene rearrangement. At present, PRRs are categorized into four types: Toll-like receptors (TLRs), nucleotide-binding oligomerization domain (NOD)-like receptors (NLRs), RIG-I-like receptors, and C-type lectin-like receptors (Brubaker et al. 2015). These PRRs are mainly expressed on the cell surface or the cytosolic regions of innate immune cells such as antigen-presenting cells and epithelial cells. Upon microbial infection, MAMPs activate PRRs to eradicate or control microorganisms, in concert with adaptive immune responses against microbe-specific antigens. Under sterile inflammatory conditions, endogenous non-microbial danger molecules released from dying and necrotic cells activate PRRs and have been implicated in the development of autoimmune diseases (Kono and Rock 2008). Recent studies have revealed a possible involvement of MAMPs and DAMPs in the immune pathogenesis of IgG4-RD.

2.2 *IgG4-RD and MAMPs*

It is generally accepted that excessive immune reactions toward the intestinal microflora cause inflammatory bowel disease (IBD) (Bouma and Strober 2003). Indeed, significant numbers of patients with Crohn's disease present mutations in caspase recruitment domain 15 (Hugot et al. 2001; Ogura et al. 2001), which encodes NOD2, a sensor for small peptides derived from the bacterial peptidoglycan (Strober et al. 2014). NOD2 polymorphisms associated with Crohn's disease are thought to alter the immune response to gut bacteria and, consequently, the composition of the intestinal microflora (Strober et al. 2014). Thus, studies on the immune pathogenesis of Crohn's disease in the presence of NOD2 mutations have revealed an excessive immune response to MAMPs derived from the intestinal microflora.

Given the lack of definitive genome-wide association or microbiome studies on IgG4-RD, it remains to be seen whether scenario described above applies to this disorder. Some studies suggest a possible involvement of MAMPs in the development of IgG4-RD. IBD is categorized in two subsets, Crohn's disease and ulcerative colitis. The intestinal mucosa of IBD is characterized by enhanced production of TH1 cytokines, such as interleukin (IL)-12 and interferon (IFN)-γ, in Crohn's disease, and TH2 cytokines, such as IL-5 and IL-13, in ulcerative colitis (Bouma and Strober 2003). Extensive immunohistochemical analysis of IgG4-positive plasma cells in the colonic mucosa of IBD patients revealed a significantly higher number of such cells in patients with ulcerative colitis than in those with Crohn's disease (Virk et al. 2014). In addition, in ulcerative colitis, colonic infiltration of IgG4-positive plasma cells was accompanied by severe inflammation (Kuwata et al. 2014). These clinicopathological studies suggest that accumulation and infiltration of IgG4-expressing plasma cells in the colonic mucosa of patients with ulcerative colitis are probably caused by an excessive immune reaction against the intestinal microflora. Supporting this idea, Akitake et al. (2010) reported a case of IgG4-RD presenting abundant infiltration of IgG4-expressing plasmacytes in the ileum and colon without any symptoms of IBD. Furthermore, peripheral blood mononuclear cells isolated from this patient produced large amounts of TH2 cytokines upon stimulation with TLR ligands (Akitake et al. 2010). In line with this case report, the NOD2 ligand, muramyl dipeptide (MDP), has been shown to strongly induce IgG4 production in healthy individuals (Watanabe et al. 2012), which suggests that MAMPs derived from the intestinal microflora may trigger TH2-driven pathogenic responses in IgG4-RD. Repeated administration of heat-killed *Escherichia coli* to C57BL/6 mice induces activation of the innate immune system and the development of chronic fibroinflammatory disorder of the pancreas, akin to human AIP (Haruta et al. 2010; Yanagisawa et al. 2014). Taken together, both human and animal studies provide evidence that MAMPs derived from the intestinal microflora might trigger IgG4-RD through activation of PRRs.

One major question arising from the above hypothesis is whether a significant population of patients with IgG4-RD exhibits clinical symptoms of IBD. To this end, a case–control study revealed that four of 71 patients with AIP had concurrent IBD (Ravi et al. 2009). The simultaneous occurrence of IBD is generally observed in patients with type 2 non-IgG4-associated AIP rather than in patients with type 1 IgG4-associated AIP (Hart et al. 2015). Moreover, Ueki et al. (2015) reported an extremely low incidence of AIP in patients with IBD (Ueki et al. 2015). Thus, previous case–control studies do not support the hypothesis that MAMPs derived from the intestinal microflora are involved in the development of IgG4-RD. Given that intestinal tissue injury is absent even in the presence of massive infiltration of IgG4-expressing plasma cells (Akitake et al. 2010), the underlying immune reactions do not play a pathogenic role in the gut. In this regard, several mechanisms, including Tregs-mediated immune suppression, might protect the intestinal mucosa from tissue injury (Strober et al. 2007). Thus, one possible explanation for the low incidence of IBD in IgG4-RD patients is that pathogenic immune responses leading to colonic injury are suppressed by activation of Tregs. In contrast, these responses might cause tissue injury in sterile organs, such as the pancreas and salivary glands, due to the absence of regulatory mechanisms. Future studies addressing global immune reactions in the gut mucosa of patients with AIP will confirm this hypothesis.

2.3 *IgG4-RD and DAMPs*

DAMPs released from dying or necrotic cells are now recognized as potent activators of the innate immune system (Kono and Rock 2008). The role of DAMPs is highlighted in acute pancreatitis (Hoque et al. 2011, 2012). Double-stranded DNA (dsDNA) released from dying acinar cells upon experimental induction of acute pancreatitis activates TLR9 and NLR family, pyrin domain-containing 3 (NLRP3). These receptors are expressed in antigen-presenting cells and stimulate production of proinflammatory cytokines, such as IL-1β and IL-18 (Hoque et al. 2011, 2012). High-mobility group box chromosomal protein 1 (HMGB1) is a well-studied DAMP capable of inducing sterile inflammation by activating TLR4 (Zong et al. 2013). Yasuda et al. (2006) reported a marked increase in serum levels of HMGB1 in patients with acute pancreatitis. These studies support the idea that DAMPs released from necrotic pancreatic tissues induce the development of acute pancreatitis through activation of the innate immune system. Similarly, several reports suggest the involvement of DAMPs, such as dsDNA, monosodium urate crystals (MSU), and asbestos in the pathogenesis of IgG4-RD. Serum levels of dsDNA are higher in patients with IgG4-RD than in those with chronic pancreatitis or healthy individuals (Arai et al. 2015). Antigen-presenting cells and neutrophils isolated from patients with IgG4-RD induce IgG4 production by B cells upon MSU stimulation (Arai et al. 2015). Furthermore, Toyoshima et al. (2010) reported a case of IgG4-related lung disease in a worker exposed to asbestos, one of the prototypical DAMPs to activate the NLRP3 inflammasome (Toyoshima et al. 2010). It should nevertheless be noted that our knowledge of DAMPs in IgG4-RD is very limited and definitive proof is still lacking at present.

3 IgG4-RD and T Helper Type 2 Cytokines

Lesions in patients with IgG4-RD are characterized by enhanced expression of TH2 cytokines, such as IL-4, IL-10, and IL-13, rather than TH1 cytokines, such as IFN-γ and IL-12 (Della-Torre et al. 2015; Moriyama et al. 2014; Tanaka et al. 2012). In vitro studies have shown that stimulation of peripheral blood mononuclear cells with IL-4 and/or IL-10 increases IgG4 production in healthy subjects (Jeannin et al. 1998; Punnonen et al. 1993). The involvement of TH2 cytokines partly explains the allergic symptoms and elevated serum IgE levels commonly detected in IgG4-RD patients. It should be noted, however, that such classical TH2 responses might play a pathogenic role only in a defined subpopulation of IgG4-RD. Expansion of cells expressing IL-4, IL-5, or IL-13 and their lineage transcription factor GATA binding protein 3 (GATA3) (Crotty 2014) has been detected only in IgG4-RD patients with atopic symptoms and not in those without these symptoms (Mattoo et al. 2014a). Co-localization analyses on cells expressing both GATA3 and IL-4, IL-5, or IL-13 have not been performed in the lesions of IgG4-RD patients. Therefore, it is possible that IL-4 and IL-13 may be derived from other types of cells, such as T follicular helper (Tfh) cells (Akiyama et al. 2015; Maehara et al. 2012; Moriyama et al. 2014) and mast cells (Takeuchi et al. 2014, 2015) rather than conventional TH2 cells.

Tfh is a newly defined T helper subset that induces the development of germinal centers and the generation of high-affinity antibodies by B cells (Crotty 2014). Tfh cells express the master transcription factor B cell lymphoma 6 (Bcl6) and the chemokine receptor CXCR5 and produce large amounts of IL-21 (Crotty 2014). Maehara et al. (2012) reported increased IL-21 and BCL6 expression in the ectopic germinal centers of salivary glands from a patient with IgG4-RD (Maehara et al. 2012). Furthermore, flow cytometric analysis by Akiyama et al. (2015) found elevated numbers of $CXCR5^+$ $CD45RA^-$ $CD4^+$ $CXCR3^-$ $CCR6^-$ Tfh2 cells in the peripheral blood of IgG4-RD patients. Interestingly, the number of Tfh2 cells correlated with IL-4 and IgG4 serum levels, suggesting that Tfh cells may enhance the production of IgG4 in concert with conventional TH2 cells.

Another important feature of the T cell subset in IgG4-RD is infiltration of Tregs in the lesions (Miyoshi et al. 2008; Zen et al. 2007). Tregs express the master transcription factor, forkhead box protein p3 (Foxp3), and produce immunosuppressive cytokines, such as IL-10 and tumor growth factor (TGF)-β1 (Morikawa and Sakaguchi 2014), as observed in the liver of IgG4-RD patients (Zen et al. 2007). In vitro studies have shown that Tregs induce IgG4 production by B cells through IL-10 and TGF-β1 (Satoguina et al. 2008). Thus, it is likely that Tregs-derived IL-10 and TGF-β1 are associated with enhanced IgG4 production. One major question concerns the mechanism underlying the occurrence of chronic inflammation even in the presence of Tregs in IgG4-RD. In this regard, it should be noted that no studies have addressed the function of Tregs isolated from IgG4-RD patients by using conventional suppression assays. This leaves the possibility that Tregs accumulating in the lesions of IgG4-RD patients cannot fulfill their suppressive activity due to impaired immune regulatory functions, thus leading to chronic fibroinflammatory disorders. Alternatively, activation of Tregs in IgG4-RD may reflect some sort of counter-regulatory response to strong and persistent inflammation.

As suggested above, adaptive immune responses associated with IgG4-RD are mediated by a variety of T cell subsets, including classical TH2 cells, Tfh cells, and Tregs. Even if the elevated cytokine expression observed in IgG4-RD is confirmed to be derived from these T cell subsets, further studies are required to elucidate the cellular and molecular mechanisms accounting for pathological adaptive immune responses.

4 T Cell-Independent IgG4 Production (Fig. 1)

Innate immune responses mediated by MAMPs and DAMPs may be important for the onset and maintenance of abnormal immunological environments leading to IgG4-RD. Watanabe et al. (2012) have addressed the role of TLR- or NLR-mediated signaling pathways in the production of IgG4, and some key findings are summarized herein (Watanabe et al. 2012, 2013). First, MDP was found to be a potent inducer of IgG4 production (Watanabe et al. 2012). Second, MDP activation of NOD2 in monocytes induced the production of B cell-activating factor (BAFF), thereby enhancing IgG4 production through inhibition of B cell apoptosis. These results were obtained from peripheral blood mononuclear cells (PBMCs) of healthy subjects, suggesting the importance of NOD2 activation for IgG4 production in innate immune cells. Third, PBMCs isolated from IgG4-RD patients produced large amounts of IgG4 and BAFF upon stimulation with TLR and NLR ligands. Finally, B cells from healthy controls produced large quantities of IgG4 upon stimulation with TLR and NLR ligands via a T cell-independent manner only when co-cultured with monocytes isolated from patients with IgG4-RD. These results suggest that activation of the innate immune system by TLR and NLR ligands may be a critical step for the increased production of IgG4 and that IgG4 production can be induced without any help by T cells (Watanabe et al. 2012). As for the molecular mechanism accounting for BAFF production, involvement of

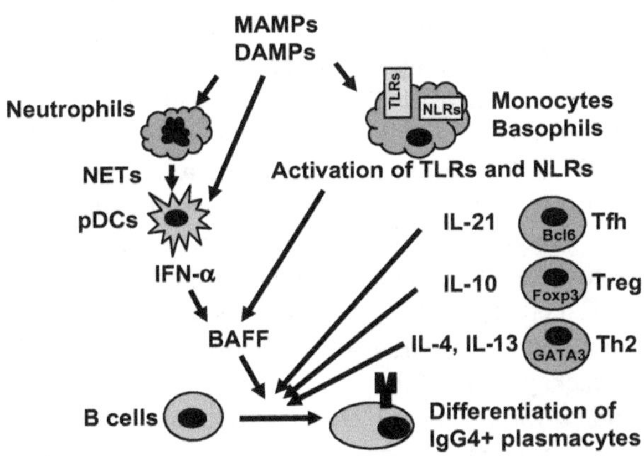

Fig. 1 Innate immune responses associated with IgG4-RD. Damage-associated molecular patterns (*DAMPs*) and microbe-associated molecular patterns (*MAMPs*) activate innate immune receptors, such as Toll-like receptors (*TLRs*) and NOD-like receptors (*NLRs*) expressed in plasmacytoid dendritic cells (*pDCs*), monocytes, and basophils. Activation of pDCs by neutrophil extracellular traps (*NETs*) leads to robust production of IFN-α and BAFF, whereas activation of TLRs and NLRs leads to robust production of BAFF. IgG4 production by B cells is enhanced upon co-culture with pDCs, monocytes, and basophils in a T cell-independent manner. Additionally, regulatory T (*Treg*), T helper type 2 (*Th2*), and T follicular helper (*Tfh*) cells stimulate IgG4 production by B cells through IL-4, IL-10, IL-13, and IL-21

NF-κB activation has been suggested. Inhibition of NF-κB signaling pathways reduces BAFF production by monocytes upon stimulation with MDP (Watanabe et al. 2012). Moreover, the DNA sequence of the BAFF promoter has several functional binding motifs for the NF-κB subunit (He et al. 2003).

Although basophils have been considered effector cells for TH2 and IgE responses, recent studies have highlighted their role in initiating allergic responses (Paul and Zhu 2010; Sokol and Medzhitov 2010). It seems likely that activation of basophils is involved in the immune pathogenesis of IgG4-RD, which is often characterized by elevated serum IgE levels. Indeed, Watanabe et al. (2013) showed that activation of TLRs in basophils stimulated IgG4 production by B cells in a T cell-independent manner (Watanabe et al. 2013). Basophils were found to release large quantities of BAFF upon stimulation with TLR ligands, thereby triggering IgG4 production. More importantly, as with monocytes (Watanabe et al. 2012), it was shown that B cells from healthy controls produced considerable amounts of IgG4 upon stimulation with TLR and NLR ligands only when co-cultured with basophils from IgG4-RD patients. These two studies suggest that activation of TLRs and/or NLRs in monocytes or basophils induces IgG4 production by B cells in a T cell-independent but BAFF-dependent manner. Moreover, monocytes or basophils from IgG4-RD patients produce large quantities of BAFF upon exposure to MAMPs via NF-κB signaling pathways.

Consistent with the above in vitro studies (Watanabe et al. 2012, 2013), BAFF serum levels are significantly higher in IgG4-RD patients than in healthy controls or in patients with chronic pancreatitis or pancreatic cancer (Kiyama et al. 2012; Yamanishi et al. 2011). Interestingly, BAFF-mediated signaling pathways seem to be operating in the inflamed pancreas, as confirmed by expression of BAFF and BAFF receptors in cells infiltrating the pancreas of IgG4-related AIP (Yamanishi et al. 2011). In addition, IgD^+ B cells stimulated with BAFF and IL-4 induce Ig class-switch DNA recombination (CSR), giving rise to IgG1, IgG2, IgG3, and IgG4 (Litinskiy et al. 2002). Taken together, these reports have identified BAFF and TH2 cytokines derived from antigen-presenting cells and T cells, respectively, to be responsible for the generation of pathogenic immune responses in IgG4-RD. It should be noted, however, that enhanced IgG4 responses in IgG4-RD cannot be explained by BAFF-mediated pathways alone, since BAFF is a survival and activation factor for B cells rather than a specific inducer for IgG4 CSR (Mackay and Schneider 2009; Mackay et al. 2007).

The above studies on IgG4 and BAFF production in response to MAMPs support the idea that commensal flora-mediated innate immunity is involved in the immunopathogenesis of IgG4-RD. In this scenario, tissue injury initiated by an autoimmune process leads to impaired gut barrier function, followed by entry of intestinal microflora into the splanchnic vascular bed. MAMPs derived from intestinal microflora activate tissue-residing antigen-presenting cells and B cells, thus stimulating production of BAFF and IgG4. This idea is consistent with the observation that IgG4-expressing plasma cells are sometimes seen in the intestinal mucosa of patients with IgG4-RD (Akitake et al. 2010; Deheragoda et al. 2007).

5 IgG4-RD and Type I IFN (Fig. 1)

Type I IFNs (IFN-α and IFN-β) are indispensable components of host defenses against viral and bacterial infections (Akira and Takeda 2004). Although rapid induction of type I IFN production is particularly beneficial against viral infections, persistent and excessive release of these pluripotent cytokines causes autoimmune diseases. Detailed and extensive studies using clinical samples from lupus patients have established that excessive production of type I IFN and activation of downstream signaling pathways play a central role in the immune pathogenesis of the disease (Crow 2014a, b; Huang et al. 2015). This was confirmed by enhanced expression of type I IFN-related genes in peripheral blood mononuclear cells from lupus patients (Baechler et al. 2003; Bennett et al. 2003). Since they produce large quantities of IFN-α (Gilliet et al. 2008), plasmacytoid dendritic cells (pDCs) are considered the main promoters of type I IFN signaling pathways in lupus (Crow 2014a, b; Huang et al. 2015). This is particularly true, if they are exposed to immune complexes containing nucleic acids (Crow 2014a, b). Thus, the innate immune response mediated by pDC-derived IFN-α plays a predominant role in the initiation and progression of lupus. This notion is supported by recent genome-wide association studies, which have identified type I IFN-related genes as susceptible loci for lupus (Deng and Tsao 2010).

A recent study by Arai et al. (2015) provides evidence that activation of pDCs and IFN-α production are prominent features of human IgG4-RD and an experimental model of AIP (Arai et al. 2015). MRL/MpJ mice treated with polyinosinic–polycytidylic acid, poly (I:C), exhibit several histological features of chronic autoimmune pancreatitis, such as massive destruction of acinar cell architecture, infiltration of immune cells, and fibrosis (Nishio et al. 2011; Schwaiger et al. 2014). Although human IgG4-related AIP and MRL/MpJ mice treated with poly (I:C) share important clinical findings, common abnormal immune responses have been poorly described. Cytokine and chemokine arrays of pancreatic lysates from MRL/MpJ mice treated with poly (I:C) revealed that type I IFN-related chemokines, such as chemokine (C-X-C motif) ligand (CXCL) 9, 10, and 11, as wells as prototypic inflammatory cytokines, such as IL-6 and tumor necrosis factor-α, increased upon induction of experimental AIP (Arai et al. 2015). Indeed, administration of poly (I:C) led to a marked increase of IFN-α and IFN-β in the serum of MRL/MpJ mice and accumulation of pDCs in the pancreas. Since both depletion of pDCs and blockade of type I IFN signaling pathways prevent pancreatic inflammation, Arai et al. (2015) propose a pivotal role for pDC-mediated IFN-α signaling pathways in experimental AIP (Arai et al. 2015). In line with the above results, serum levels of IFN-α are significantly higher in patients with IgG4-associated AIP than in healthy controls, or in patients with chronic pancreatitis (Arai et al. 2015). Consistent with a report showing that BAFF expression is directly induced by type I IFN via interferon regulatory factors 1 and 2 (Sjöstrand et al. 2016), elevated IFN-α serum levels are accompanied by BAFF levels. Moreover, infiltration of pDCs producing both IFN-α and BAFF is observed in the pancreas of patients with

IgG4-associated AIP, but not in those with chronic pancreatitis (Arai et al. 2015). Regarding activators of pDCs, two recent studies show that neutrophil extracellular traps (NETs) containing self-DNA and neutrophil-derived proteins are potent inducers of IFN-α production by pDCs in patients with lupus (Garcia-Romo et al. 2011; Lande et al. 2011). In the case of IgG4-RD, NETs may also be involved in increased IFN-α release by pDCs. Arai et al. (2015) report that B cells isolated from healthy individuals produce large quantities of IgG4 when co-cultured with NET-stimulated pDCs isolated from patients with IgG4-RD. Such pDC-mediated IgG4 production by B cells is markedly suppressed by the abrogation of type I IFN signaling pathways, which suggests an important role by pDC-derived IFN-α. Taken together, these results strongly indicate that pDC activation, followed by IFN-α release, is one of the pathogenic immune responses associated with IgG4-RD.

The study described above provides a new insight into the pathogenesis of IgG4-RD, which, like lupus, is characterized by pDC activation and IFN-α production. In addition, autoimmune complexes released by NETs may function as potent activators of pDCs in both immune disorders. Nevertheless, it should be noted that clinicopathological features of IgG4-RD and lupus are completely different, with augmented IgG4 production and storiform fibrosis being observed only in IgG4-RD. Therefore, it is clear that the immunopathogenesis of IgG4-RD cannot be explained solely by pDC activation and ensuing IFN-α production. Future studies aiming to identify immune responses other than the pDC-mediated IFN-α signaling pathways will elucidate the immunopathogenesis of IgG4-RD and help distinguish it from lupus at a cellular and a molecular level.

6 Conclusions

IgG4-RD is a newly established disease first proposed by Japanese gastroenterologists and rheumatologists. Although IgG4-RD is characterized by an adaptive response by B cells, recent studies suggest possible involvement of the innate immune system. Expression of IFN-α and BAFF produced by innate immune cells is enhanced in the pancreas of IgG4-RD patients and experimental AIP. Furthermore, pDCs and monocytes isolated from IgG4-RD patients induce a marked increase in IgG4 production by B cells through IFN-α and BAFF, respectively. Although many questions remain to be addressed, these insights into the role of innate immune responses in IgG4-RD pathogenesis support the idea that patients with IgG4-RD can be treated with inhibitors of innate immune cytokines, such as IFN-α and BAFF.

Acknowledgments This work was supported by Grant-in-Aid for Scientific Research (25293172, 15K15370) from the Japan Society for the Promotion of Science; the Kato Memorial Trust for Nambyo Research; and the Health and Labor Sciences Research Grants for Research on Intractable Diseases from the Ministry of Health, Labor and Welfare, Japan.

References

Akira S, Takeda K (2004) Toll-like receptor signalling. Nat Rev Immunol 4:499–511
Akitake R, Watanabe T, Zaima C, Uza N, Ida H, Tada S, Nishida N, Chiba T (2010) Possible involvement of T helper type 2 responses to Toll-like receptor ligands in IgG4-related sclerosing disease. Gut 59:542–545
Akiyama M, Suzuki K, Yamaoka K, Yasuoka H, Takeshita M, Kaneko Y, Kondo H, Kassai Y, Miyazaki T, Morita R et al (2015) Number of circulating follicular helper 2 T cells correlates with IgG4 and Interleukin-4 levels and plasmablast numbers in IgG4-related disease. Arthritis Rheumatol 67:2476–2481
Arai Y, Yamashita K, Kuriyama K, Shiokawa M, Kodama Y, Sakurai T, Mizugishi K, Uchida K, Kadowaki N, Takaori-Kondo A et al (2015) Plasmacytoid dendritic cell activation and IFN-alpha production are prominent features of murine autoimmune pancreatitis and human IgG4-related autoimmune pancreatitis. J Immunol 195:3033–3044
Baechler EC, Batliwalla FM, Karypis G, Gaffney PM, Ortmann WA, Espe KJ, Shark KB, Grande WJ, Hughes KM, Kapur V et al (2003) Interferon-inducible gene expression signature in peripheral blood cells of patients with severe lupus. Proc Natl Acad Sci USA 100:2610–2615
Bennett L, Palucka AK, Arce E, Cantrell V, Borvak J, Banchereau J, Pascual V (2003) Interferon and granulopoiesis signatures in systemic lupus erythematosus blood. J Exp Med 197:711–723
Bouma G, Strober W (2003) The immunological and genetic basis of inflammatory bowel disease. Nat Rev Immunol 3:521–533
Brubaker SW, Bonham KS, Zanoni I, Kagan JC (2015) Innate immune pattern recognition: a cell biological perspective. Annu Rev Immunol 33:257–290
Carruthers MN, Topazian MD, Khosroshahi A, Witzig TE, Wallace ZS, Hart PA, Deshpande V, Smyrk TC, Chari S, Stone JH (2015) Rituximab for IgG4-related disease: a prospective, open-label trial. Ann Rheum Dis 74:1171–1177
Chen G, Shaw MH, Kim YG, Nunez G (2009) NOD-like receptors: role in innate immunity and inflammatory disease. Annu Rev Pathol 4:365–398
Crotty S (2014) T follicular helper cell differentiation, function, and roles in disease. Immunity 41:529–542
Crow MK (2014a) Advances in understanding the role of type I interferons in systemic lupus erythematosus. Curr Opin Rheumatol 26:467–474
Crow MK (2014b) Type I interferon in the pathogenesis of lupus. J Immunol 192:5459–5468
Deheragoda MG, Church NI, Rodriguez-Justo M, Munson P, Sandanayake N, Seward EW, Miller K, Novelli M, Hatfield AR, Pereira SP, Webster GJ (2007) The use of immunoglobulin G4 immunostaining in diagnosing pancreatic and extrapancreatic involvement in autoimmune pancreatitis. Clin Gastroenterol Hepatol 5:1229–1234
Della-Torre E, Lanzillotta M, Doglioni C (2015) Immunology of IgG4-related disease. Clin Exp Immunol 181:191–206
Deng Y, Tsao BP (2010) Genetic susceptibility to systemic lupus erythematosus in the genomic era. Nat Rev Rheumatol 6:683–692
Fukui Y, Uchida K, Sakaguchi Y, Fukui T, Nishio A, Shikata N, Sakaida N, Uemura Y, Satoi S, Okazaki K (2015) Possible involvement of Toll-like receptor 7 in the development of type 1 autoimmune pancreatitis. J Gastroenterol 50:435–444
Garcia-Romo GS, Caielli S, Vega B, Connolly J, Allantaz F, Xu Z, Punaro M, Baisch J, Guiducci C, Coffman RL et al (2011) Netting neutrophils are major inducers of type I IFN production in pediatric systemic lupus erythematosus. Sci Transl Med 3:73ra20
Gilliet M, Cao W, Liu YJ (2008) Plasmacytoid dendritic cells: sensing nucleic acids in viral infection and autoimmune diseases. Nat Rev Immunol 8:594–606
Hamano H, Kawa S, Horiuchi A, Unno H, Furuya N, Akamatsu T, Fukushima M, Nikaido T, Nakayama K, Usuda N, Kiyosawa K (2001) High serum IgG4 concentrations in patients with sclerosing pancreatitis. N Engl J Med 344:732–738

Hart PA, Zen Y, Chari ST (2015) Recent advances in autoimmune pancreatitis. Gastroenterology 149:39–51

Haruta I, Yanagisawa N, Kawamura S, Furukawa T, Shimizu K, Kato H, Kobayashi M, Shiratori K, Yagi J (2010) A mouse model of autoimmune pancreatitis with salivary gland involvement triggered by innate immunity via persistent exposure to avirulent bacteria. Lab Invest 90:1757–1769

He B, Raab-Traub N, Casali P, Cerutti A (2003) EBV-encoded latent membrane protein 1 cooperates with BAFF/BLyS and APRIL to induce T cell-independent Ig heavy chain class switching. J Immunol 171:5215–5224

Hoque R, Sohail M, Malik A, Sarwar S, Luo Y, Shah A, Barrat F, Flavell R, Gorelick F, Husain S, Mehal W (2011) TLR9 and the NLRP3 inflammasome link acinar cell death with inflammation in acute pancreatitis. Gastroenterology 141:358–369

Hoque R, Malik AF, Gorelick F, Mehal WZ (2012) Sterile inflammatory response in acute pancreatitis. Pancreas 41:353–357

Huang X, Dorta-Estremera S, Yao Y, Shen N, Cao W (2015) Predominant role of plasmocytoid dendritic cells in stimulating systemic autoimmunity. Front Immunol 6:526

Hugot JP, Chamaillard M, Zouali H, Lesage S, Cezard JP, Belaiche J, Almer S, Tysk C, O'Morain CA, Gassull M et al (2001) Association of NOD2 leucine-rich repeat variants with susceptibility to Crohn's disease. Nature 411:599–603

Jeannin P, Lecoanet S, Delneste Y, Gauchat JF, Bonnefoy JY (1998) IgE versus IgG4 production can be differentially regulated by IL-10. J Immunol 160:3555–3561

Kamisawa T, Okamoto A (2006) Autoimmune pancreatitis: proposal of IgG4-related sclerosing disease. J Gastroenterol 41:613–625

Khosroshahi A, Bloch DB, Deshpande V, Stone JH (2010) Rituximab therapy leads to rapid decline of serum IgG4 levels and prompt clinical improvement in IgG4-related systemic disease. Arthritis Rheum 62:1755–1762

Kiyama K, Kawabata D, Hosono Y, Kitagori K, Yukawa N, Yoshifuji H, Omura K, Fujii T, Mimori T (2012) Serum BAFF and APRIL levels in patients with IgG4-related disease and their clinical significance. Arthritis Res Ther 14:R86

Kono H, Rock KL (2008) How dying cells alert the immune system to danger. Nat Rev Immunol 8:279–289

Kuwata G, Kamisawa T, Koizumi K, Tabata T, Hara S, Kuruma S, Fujiwara T, Chiba K, Egashira H, Fujiwara J et al (2014) Ulcerative colitis and immunoglobulin G4. Gut Liver 8:29–34

Lande R, Ganguly D, Facchinetti V, Frasca L, Conrad C, Gregorio J, Meller S, Chamilos G, Sebasigari R, Riccieri V et al (2011). Neutrophils activate plasmacytoid dendritic cells by releasing self-DNA-peptide complexes in systemic lupus erythematosus. Sci Transl Med 3:73ra19

Litinskiy MB, Nardelli B, Hilbert DM, He B, Schaffer A, Casali P, Cerutti A (2002) DCs induce CD40-independent immunoglobulin class switching through BLyS and APRIL. Nat Immunol 3:822–829

Mackay F, Schneider P (2009) Cracking the BAFF code. Nat Rev Immunol 9:491–502

Mackay F, Silveira PA, Brink R (2007) B cells and the BAFF/APRIL axis: fast-forward on autoimmunity and signaling. Curr Opin Immunol 19:327–336

Maehara T, Moriyama M, Nakashima H, Miyake K, Hayashida JN, Tanaka A, Shinozaki S, Kubo Y, Nakamura S (2012) Interleukin-21 contributes to germinal centre formation and immunoglobulin G4 production in IgG4-related dacryoadenitis and sialoadenitis, so-called Mikulicz's disease. Ann Rheum Dis 71:2011–2019

Masaki Y, Dong L, Kurose N, Kitagawa K, Morikawa Y, Yamamoto M, Takahashi H, Shinomura Y, Imai K, Saeki T et al (2009) Proposal for a new clinical entity, IgG4-positive multiorgan lymphoproliferative syndrome: analysis of 64 cases of IgG4-related disorders. Ann Rheum Dis 68:1310–1315

Mattoo H, Della-Torre E, Mahajan VS, Stone JH, Pillai S (2014a) Circulating Th2 memory cells in IgG4-related disease are restricted to a defined subset of subjects with atopy. Allergy 69:399–402

Mattoo H, Mahajan VS, Della-Torre E, Sekigami Y, Carruthers M, Wallace ZS, Deshpande V, Stone JH, Pillai S (2014b) De novo oligoclonal expansions of circulating plasmablasts in active and relapsing IgG4-related disease. J Allergy Clin Immunol 134:679–687

Miyoshi H, Uchida K, Taniguchi T, Yazumi S, Matsushita M, Takaoka M, Okazaki K (2008) Circulating naïve and CD4+ CD25high regulatory T cells in patients with autoimmune pancreatitis. Pancreas 36:133–140

Morikawa H, Sakaguchi S (2014) Genetic and epigenetic basis of Treg cell development and function: from a FoxP3-centered view to an epigenome-defined view of natural Treg cells. Immunol Rev 259:192–205

Moriyama M, Tanaka A, Maehara T, Furukawa S, Nakashima H, Nakamura S (2014) T helper subsets in Sjögren's syndrome and IgG4-related dacryoadenitis and sialoadenitis: a critical review. J Autoimmun 51:81–88

Nishio A, Asada M, Uchida K, Fukui T, Chiba T, Okazaki K (2011) The role of innate immunity in the pathogenesis of experimental autoimmune pancreatitis in mice. Pancreas 40:95–102

Ogura Y, Bonen DK, Inohara N, Nicolae DL, Chen FF, Ramos R, Britton H, Moran T, Karaliuskas R, Duerr RH et al (2001) A frameshift mutation in *NOD2* associated with susceptibility to Crohn's disease. Nature 411:603–606

Okazaki K, Uchida K, Fukui T (2008) Recent advances in autoimmune pancreatitis: concept, diagnosis, and pathogenesis. J Gastroenterol 43:409–418

Paul WE, Zhu J (2010) How are TH2-type immune responses initiated and amplified? Nat Rev Immunol 10:225–235

Punnonen J, Aversa G, Cocks BG, McKenzie AN, Menon S, Zurawski G, de Waal Malefyt R, de Vries JE (1993) Interleukin 13 induces interleukin 4-independent IgG4 and IgE synthesis and CD23 expression by human B cells. Proc Natl Acad Sci USA 90:3730–3734

Ravi K, Chari ST, Vege SS, Sandborn WJ, Smyrk TC, Loftus EV Jr (2009) Inflammatory bowel disease in the setting of autoimmune pancreatitis. Inflamm Bowel Dis 15:1326–1330

Satoguina JS, Adjobimey T, Arndts K, Hoch J, Oldenburg J, Layland LE, Hoerauf A (2008) Tr1 and naturally occurring regulatory T cells induce IgG4 in B cells through GITR/GITR-L interaction, IL-10 and TGF-β. Eur J Immunol 38:3101–3113

Schwaiger T, van den Brandt C, Fitzner B, Zaatreh S, Kraatz F, Dummer A, Nizze H, Evert M, Broker BM, Brunner-Weinzierl MC et al (2014) Autoimmune pancreatitis in MRL/Mp mice is a T cell-mediated disease responsive to cyclosporine A and rapamycin treatment. Gut 63:494–505

Sjöstrand M, Johansson A, Aqrawi L, Olsson T, Wahren-Herlenius M, Espinosa A (2016) The expression of BAFF is controlled by IRF transcription factors. J Immunol 196:91–96

Sokol CL, Medzhitov R (2010) Emerging functions of basophils in protective and allergic immune responses. Mucosal Immunol 3:129–137

Stone JH, Zen Y, Deshpande V (2012) IgG4-related disease. N Engl J Med 366:539–551

Strober W, Murray PJ, Kitani A, Watanabe T (2006) Signalling pathways and molecular interactions of NOD1 and NOD2. Nat Rev Immunol 6:9–20

Strober W, Fuss I, Mannon P (2007) The fundamental basis of inflammatory bowel disease. J Clin Invest 117:514–521

Strober W, Asano N, Fuss I, Kitani A, Watanabe T (2014) Cellular and molecular mechanisms underlying NOD2 risk-associated polymorphisms in Crohn's disease. Immunol Rev 260:249–260

Takeuchi M, Sato Y, Ohno K, Tanaka S, Takata K, Gion Y, Orita Y, Ito T, Tachibana T, Yoshino T (2014) T helper 2 and regulatory T-cell cytokine production by mast cells: a key factor in the pathogenesis of IgG4-related disease. Mod Pathol 27:1126–1136

Takeuchi M, Ohno K, Takata K, Gion Y, Tachibana T, Orita Y, Yoshino T, Sato Y (2015) Interleukin 13-positive mast cells are increased in immunoglobulin G4-related sialadenitis. Sci Rep 5:7696

Tanaka A, Moriyama M, Nakashima H, Miyake K, Hayashida JN, Maehara T, Shinozaki S, Kubo Y, Nakamura S (2012) Th2 and regulatory immune reactions contribute to IgG4 production and the initiation of Mikulicz disease. Arthritis Rheum 64:254–263

Toyoshima M, Chida K, Kono M, Kaida Y, Nakamura Y, Suda T, Sugimura H (2010) IgG4-related lung disease in a worker occupationally exposed to asbestos. Intern Med 49:1175–1178

Ueki T, Kawamoto K, Otsuka Y, Minoda R, Maruo T, Matsumura K, Noma E, Mitsuyasu T, Otani K, Aomi Y et al (2015) Prevalence and clinicopathological features of autoimmune pancreatitis in Japanese patients with inflammatory bowel disease. Pancreas 44:434–440

Virk R, Shinagare S, Lauwers GY, Yajnik V, Stone JH, Deshpande V (2014) Tissue IgG4-positive plasma cells in inflammatory bowel disease: a study of 88 treatment-naive biopsies of inflammatory bowel disease. Mod Pathol 27:454–459

Wallace ZS, Mattoo H, Carruthers M, Mahajan VS, Della Torre E, Lee H, Kulikova M, Deshpande V, Pillai S, Stone JH (2015) Plasmablasts as a biomarker for IgG4-related disease, independent of serum IgG4 concentrations. Ann Rheum Dis 74:190–195

Watanabe T, Yamashita K, Fujikawa S, Sakurai T, Kudo M, Shiokawa M, Kodama Y, Uchida K, Okazaki K, Chiba T (2012) Activation of toll-like receptors and nucleotide-binding oligomerization domain-like receptors is involved in enhanced IgG4 responses in autoimmune pancreatitis. Arthritis Rheum 64:914–924

Watanabe T, Yamashita K, Sakurai T, Kudo M, Shiokawa M, Uza N, Kodama Y, Uchida K, Okazaki K, Chiba T (2013) Toll-like receptor activation in basophils contributes to the development of IgG4-related disease. J Gastroenterol 48:247–253

Yamanishi H, Kumagi T, Yokota T, Azemoto N, Koizumi M, Kobayashi Y, Abe M, Murakami H, Hiasa Y, Matsuura B et al (2011) Clinical significance of B cell-activating factor in autoimmune pancreatitis. Pancreas 40:840–845

Yanagisawa N, Haruta I, Shimizu K, Furukawa T, Higuchi T, Shibata N, Shiratori K, Yagi J (2014) Identification of commensal flora-associated antigen as a pathogenetic factor of autoimmune pancreatitis. Pancreatology 14:100–106

Yasuda T, Ueda T, Takeyama Y, Shinzeki M, Sawa H, Nakajima T, Ajiki T, Fujino Y, Suzuki Y, Kudoda Y (2006) Significant increase of serum high-mobility group box chromosomal protein 1 levels in patients with severe acute pancreatitis. Pancreas 33:359–363

Zen Y, Fujii T, Harada K, Kawano M, Yamada K, Takahira M, Nakanuma Y (2007) Th2 and regulatory immune reactions are increased in immunoglobin G4-related sclerosing pancreatitis and cholangitis. Hepatology 45:1538–1546

Zong M, Bruton JD, Grundtman C, Yang H, Li JH, Alexanderson H, Palmblad K, Andersson U, Harris HE, Lundberg IE, Westerblad H (2013) TLR4 as receptor for HMGB1 induced muscle dysfunction in myositis. Ann Rheum Dis 72:1390–1399

Kolibri 360 GmbH
Ferdinand-Jühlke-Straße 7
99095 Erfurt, Deutschland
produktsicherheit@kolibri360.de